An Atlas of Investigation and Management
ASTHMA

An Atlas of Investigation and Management

ASTHMA

Sebastian L Johnston MBBS, PhD, FRCP
Professor of Respiratory Medicine
Department of Respiratory Medicine
National Heart and Lung Institute
Wright Fleming Institute of Infection and Immunity
MRC and Asthma UK Centre in Allergic Mechanisms of Asthma
Imperial College London
London, UK

CLINICAL PUBLISHING
OXFORD

Clinical Publishing
an imprint of Atlas Medical Publishing Ltd
Oxford Centre for Innovation
Mill Street, Oxford OX2 0JX, UK

Tel: +44 1865 811116
Fax: +44 1865 251550
Email: info@clinicalpublishing.co.uk
Web: www.clinicalpublishing.co.uk

Distributed in USA and Canada by:
Clinical Publishing
30 Amberwood Parkway
Ashland OH 44805 USA

Tel: 800-247-6553 (toll free within U.S. and Canada)
Fax: 419-281-6883
Email: order@bookmasters.com

Distributed in UK and Rest of World by:
Marston Book Services Ltd
PO Box 269
Abingdon
Oxon OX14 4YN UK

Tel: +44 1235 465500
Fax: +44 1235 465555
Email: trade.orders@marston.co.uk

A catalogue record of this book is available from the British Library

ISBN-13 978 1 904392 18 7
ISBN-10 1 904392 18 0

**The publisher makes no representation, express or implied, that the dosages
in this book are correct. Readers must therefore always check the product
information and clinical procedures with the most up-to-date published product
information and data sheets provided by the manufacturers and the most recent
codes of conduct and safety regulations. The authors and the publisher do not
accept any liability for any errors in the text or for the misuse or misapplication
of material in this work.**

Project manager: Gavin Smith, GPS Publishing Solutions, Herts, UK
Typeset by Phoenix Photosetting, Chatham, Kent, UK
Printed by T G Hostench SA, Barcelona, Spain

Contents

Contributors

Mubarak Alajmi, MD, D-ABIM, FRCPC
Specialist in Pulmonary Medicine
Respiratory Unit
Department of Medicine
Al-Adan Hospital
Kuwait

Sarah Aldington, BMedSci, BMBS, MRCP(UK)
Senior Research Fellow
Medical Research Institute of New Zealand
Wellington
New Zealand

Richard Beasley, MBChB, FRACP, DM, FAAAAI, FRCP, DSc
Respiratory Physician
Medical Research Institute of New Zealand
Wellington
New Zealand

Nasser Behbehani, MB, BCh, FRCPC
Associate Professor
Department of Medicine
Kuwait University
Kuwait

Liz Biggart, MSc, RSCN
Children's Respiratory Nurse Specialist
Department of Paediatric Respiratory Medicine
Royal Brompton Hospital
London
UK

Peter Burney, MA, MD, FRCP, FFPH, FMedSci
Professor of Respiratory Epidemiology and Public Health
National Heart and Lung Institute
Imperial College
London
UK

Andrew Bush, MD, FRCP, FRCPCH
Professor of Paediatric Respirology
Department of Paediatric Respiratory Medicine
Royal Brompton Hospital
London
UK

Chris J. Corrigan, MA, MSc, PhD, FRCP
Department of Asthma, Allergy and Respiratory Science
Guy's Hospital
London
UK

Gwyneth A. Davies, MB, BCh, MRCP
Lecturer in Medicine
School of Medicine
Swansea University
Swansea
Wales

J. Mark FitzGerald, MB, MD, FRCPI, FRCPC
Director Centre for Clinical Epidemiology and Evaluation,
Vancouver Coastal Health Research Institute
Professor of Medicine,
Head, UBC and VGH Division of Respiratory Medicine
Vancouver
British Columbia
Canada

Pranab Haldar, MA, MRCP
Specialist Registrar, Respiratory Medicine
Department of Respiratory Medicine
Glenfield Hospital
Leicester
UK

Julian M. Hopkin, MD, MSc, MA, FRCP, FRCPE, FMedSci
Professor of Medicine
School of Medicine
Swansea University
Swansea
Wales

Nikolaos G. Papadopoulos, MD, PhD
Lecturer in Pediatric Allergy
Research Laboratories
"P & A Kyriakou" Children's Hospital
Second Department of Pediatrics
University of Athens
Athens
Greece

Ian D. Pavord, DM, FRCP
Consultant Physician and Honorary Professor of Medicine
Department of Respiratory Medicine
Glenfield Hospital
Leicester
UK

Cesar Picado, MD, PhD
Senior Consultant in Pneumology
Professor of Medicine
Department of Respiratory Medicine
Hospital Clinic
University of Barcelona
Barcelona
Spain

Sejal Saglani, BSc, MBChB, MRCPCH, MD
Senior Lecturer in Respiratory Paediatrics
Department of Paediatric Respiratory Medicine
Royal Brompton Hospital
London
UK

Dominick Shaw, MB ChB, MRCP
Specialist Registrar, Respiratory Medicine
Department of Respiratory Medicine and Thoracic Surgery
Glenfield Hospital
Leicester
UK

Chrysanthi L. Skevaki, MD
Lecturer in Pediatric Allergy
Research Laboratories
"P & A Kyriakou" Children's Hospital
Second Department of Pediatrics
University of Athens
Athens
Greece

Nick H. T. ten Hacken, MD, PhD
Associate Professor of Pulmonology
Department of Pulmonology
University Medical Center and University of Groningen
The Netherlands

Wim Timens, MD, PhD
Professor of Pathology
Department of Pathology
University Medical Center and University of Groningen
The Netherlands

Preface

Asthma is an increasingly common chronic respiratory condition, which now affects 1 in 3 children and 1 in 5 adults in westernised countries. Over the past 20–30 years, we have begun to understand a good deal about asthma, and the same time frame has seen considerable advances in its treatment. However, much remains to be learned and there remain many asthmatics who are undiagnosed and many that are diagnosed are under-treated. Acute exacerbations are the major cause of morbidity, mortality and healthcare costs associated with asthma – regrettably they continue to occur despite best use of currently available therapies indicating that new approaches to therapy are still needed. Severe asthma is another significant factor contributing to morbidity and increased healthcare costs and this too is inadequately treated by currently available therapies. The importance of asthma and the constantly emerging new knowledge regarding its pathogenesis and treatment requires constant updating of the literature available in order to keep us as well informed as possible. It is therefore timely to bring together world experts on asthma to summarise our current state of knowledge in an easy-to-access format – an atlas, in which pictorial representations are accompanied by explanatory text to maximise readability and accessibility of the information contained therein.

The definition and diagnosis of asthma remain a challenge: with related but different disease phenotypes being recognised, and many cases being unrecognised, these subjects thus form the starting point of this atlas. The epidemiology, clinical types of asthma and the aetiology are also interconnected and vitally important subjects, with epidemiology providing important clues to the aetiology, aetiology determining clinical types and the clinical types being essential for accurate epidemiology. One classical phenotype of severe asthma is Churg–Strauss syndrome, which is described in detail with clinical cases for illustration. Next, the pathophysiology of asthma is described, followed appropriately by treatment and prevention strategies for both stable asthma and acute exacerbations. Finally, as the population most afflicted by this disease, we have a separate chapter dedicated to asthma in children.

My sincere and grateful thanks are extended to all the contributors who gave so generously of their time and expertise in putting this atlas together. I hope very much that you find the contents stimulating and informative and that this volume will provoke further efforts to research the aetiology and pathogenesis of asthma that will lead eventually to the development of new treatments to more effectively prevent and treat this often debilitating condition.

Sebastian L. Johnston, MBBS, PhD, FRCP
February 2007

Abbreviations

ANCA	antineutrophilic cytoplasmic antibody
AP	activator protein
BHR	bronchial hyper-responsiveness
BMI	body mass index
COX	cyclo-oxygenase
CSS	Churg–Strauss syndrome
CT	computed tomography
ECRHS	European Community Respiratory Health Survey
ERK	extracellular signal-regulated protein kinase
FeNO	fractional exhaled nitric oxide
FEV_1	forced expiratory volume in one second
FVC	forced vital capacity
GMCSF	granulocyte macrophage colony stimulating factor
GOR	gastro-oesophageal reflux
HLA	human leucocyte antigen
IFV	influenza virus
IL	interleukin
INF	interferon
LABA	long acting β-agonist
MAP	mitogen-activated protein
MEK	mitogen-activated or extracellular signal-regulated protein kinase
NSAID	non-steroidal anti-inflammatory drug
PAF	platelet-activating factor
PCR	polymerase chain reaction
PEFR	peak expiratory flow rate
PG	prostaglandin
PIV	parainfluenza virus
pMDI	pressurized metered dose inhaler
PP	pulsus paradoxus
RBM	reticular basement membrane
RSV	respiratory syncytial virus
RV	rhinoviruses
SABA	short acting β-agonist
Th	T helper
TNF	tumour necrosis factor

Chapter 1

Definition and Diagnosis of Asthma

Sarah Aldington and Richard Beasley

Definition

Asthma is a lung condition that has been recognized since ancient times, with references found in ancient Egyptian, Hebrew, Greek and Indian medical writings. The word *asthma* is derived from the Greek word αστμα meaning panting or short drawn breath. It is evident from the early historical accounts of asthma that the essential clinical features were well recognized and described.

The CIBA guest symposium of 1958 proposed the following definition[1]:

widespread narrowing of the bronchial airways, which changes in severity over short periods of time either spontaneously or under treatment, and is not due to cardiovascular disease.

In the 1960s, the cardinal clinical feature of asthma, reversible airflow obstruction, formed the basis of the American Thoracic Society definition of asthma, namely that:

Asthma is a disease characterized by wide variations over short periods of time in resistance of the airways of the lung.

More recently the major clinical and physiological characteristics of asthma have been incorporated in an operational definition which also recognizes the underlying disease mechanisms. In this way the recent Global Initiative for Asthma guidelines[2] state that:

Asthma is a chronic inflammatory disorder of the airways in which many cells and cellular elements play a role. The chronic inflammation causes an associated increase in airway hyperresponsiveness that leads to recurrent episodes of wheezing, breathlessness, chest tightness and coughing, particularly at night or in the early morning. These episodes are usually associated with widespread but variable airflow obstruction that is often reversible either spontaneously or with treatment.

These three components – chronic airways inflammation, enhanced bronchial responsiveness, and reversible airflow obstruction – represent the major pathophysiological events in asthma, leading to the symptoms by which the diagnosis is made.

Airways inflammation

Acute and chronic inflammation occurs in patients with different forms of asthma of differing severity[3]. The airways inflammation results in mucus plugging of the airways lumen, epithelial disruption, infiltration of the airways with eosinophils and lymphocytes, and vasodilation with microvascular

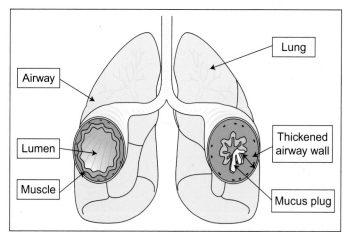

1.1 Airways in the normal state (left) and in asthma (right), demonstrating the narrowing of the airway lumen due to thickening of the airway wall and mucus plugging, which leads to a greater resistance to the flow of air in and out of the lungs. Courtesy of PK Jeffery.

leakage (**1.1**). Extensive mucus plugging often occurs in severe asthma, and it is one of the reasons bronchodilator medications have a minimal effect in this situation (**1.2**).

Airway remodelling may also occur with trophic changes such as smooth muscle hyperplasia and hypertrophy, new vessel formation, increased numbers of epithelial goblet cells and deposition of interstitial collagen beneath the epithelium (**1.3**). Recognition of the role of inflammation as the predominant disease process in asthma underlines the use of inhaled corticosteroid therapy in the long-term management of asthma, and the use of systemic corticosteroids in severe exacerbations.

Bronchial hyper-responsiveness

The enhanced sensitivity of the airways in asthma, causing bronchospasm in response to irritants that do not normally affect people without asthma is referred to as bronchial hyper-responsiveness and represents one of the basic physiological abnormalities in asthma[4] (**1.4**).

Bronchial hyper-responsiveness can be measured in the laboratory by determining the dose of constrictor agonist required to cause a specific fall in lung function (**1.5**). A wide range of constrictor agonists have been used in the measurement of bronchial responsiveness. They may be classified as causing airflow limitation directly by stimulating airway smooth muscle (e.g. methacholine or histamine), indirectly by activating mediator-secreting cells such as mast cells (e.g. exercise, cold air) or by sensory nerve stimulation (e.g. bradykinin).

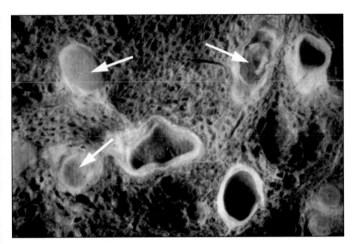

1.2 Section of a lung from a patient who died from asthma showing the occlusion of airways by mucus (arrows). Reproduced with permission from Clark T (guest ed) (1983). *Steroids in Asthma: A Reappraisal in the Light of Inhalation Therapy*. ADIS Press, Auckland.

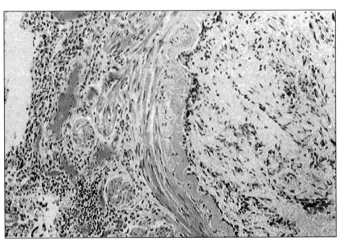

1.3 A section from the lung of a boy who died from asthma, showing inflammatory changes and airway remodelling. With permission from Clark T, Rees J (1985). *Practical Management of Asthma*. Martin Dunitz Ltd, London.

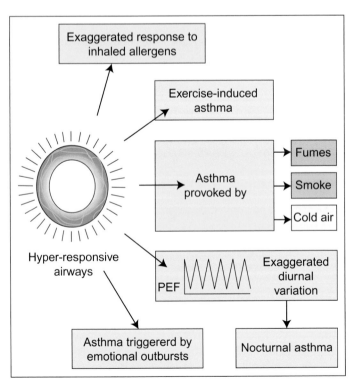

1.4 The hyper-responsive airways in asthma respond to a wide range of provoking factors. PEF, peak expiratory flow. Courtesy of ST Holgate.

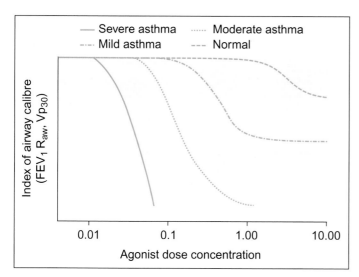

1.5 Change in the shape of the agonist/airway calibre/ dose–response characteristics for normal and asthmatic subjects according to underlying disease severity. Note the change in the maximum fall in moderate and severe asthma. R_{aw}, airways resistance; Vp_{30}, airflow at 70% of forced vital capacity measured from total lung capacity after a forced partial expiratory flow manoeuvre; FEV_1, forced expiratory volume in one second. Courtesy of ST Holgate.

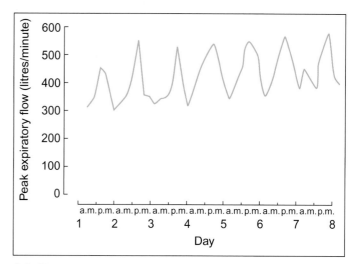

1.6 Characteristic pattern of peak flow in asthma. The peak flow record of an untreated patient with asthma shows characteristic variability, being worse in the early morning and better in the late afternoon. Courtesy of TJH Clark.

Reversible airflow obstruction

The clinical consequence of airways inflammation and bronchial hyper-responsiveness is an increased variability in airway calibre in response to provoking factors encountered in everyday life[5] (**1.6**). Reversible airflow obstruction occurring in these situations is crucial in the diagnosis of asthma as outlined below.

Diagnosis

The clinical diagnosis of asthma is usually based on an accurate history, supported by physical examination, and confirmed by the demonstration of reversible airflow obstruction with repeated measures of lung function[5].

History

The characteristic symptoms of asthma are wheezing, chest tightness, cough and breathlessness (*Table 1.1*), which are episodic and occur in response to a wide range of clinical situations and provoking factors. In diagnosis, an attempt is made to elucidate the presence of these symptoms in response to recognized provoking factors or clinical situations. The following points should be noted:

- The occurrence of wheezing is the most important symptom to support a diagnosis of asthma.
- In some individuals not all symptoms are present, or some symptoms may predominate.
- The presence and frequency of some symptoms (e.g. nocturnal wakening) may help determine disease severity.
- Some provoking factors may help to identify risk factors for the development of asthma (e.g. occupational asthma).

Examination

Physical examination may not be helpful in the diagnosis of asthma because airflow obstruction may not be present at the time of the consultation. Widespread rhonchi on auscultation of the chest should be sought; if these are not found, the patient is asked to perform a forced expiratory manoeuvre, which may provoke audible wheeze or rhonchi. Signs of differential diagnoses and other allergic disorders (e.g. eczema, rhinoconjunctivitis) should also be sought.

Objective assessment

Objective assessment of variable airflow obstruction is crucial in confirming the diagnosis of asthma (*Table 1.2*). There are

Table 1.1 Consider the diagnosis of asthma in patients with some or all of the following

Symptoms	Signs
Episodic/variable:	• None (common)
• Wheeze	• Wheeze – diffuse, bilateral, expiratory (± inspiratory)
• Shortness of breath	• Tachypnoea
• Chest tightness	
• Cough	

four methods of assessment which can be used[2, 5], with the approach chosen depending on the clinical circumstances:

- *Home peak flow monitoring* involves the repeated measurement of peak flow, before and after inhaled β-agonist, at different times of the day and night (if symptomatic) (**1.7**). Asthmatic individuals show variability of more than 20% between the highest and lowest peak flow rates, determined from pre-bronchodilator and post-bronchodilator recordings or from repeated measurements of peak flow over time; diurnal variation may also be apparent. This period of monitoring is useful not only to confirm the diagnosis of asthma, but also to determine its severity and to provide a basis for the introduction of a guided self-management plan.
- *Bronchodilator responsiveness* is determined by measuring forced expiratory volume in one second (FEV_1) or peak flow before and after administration of bronchodilator during the clinical consultation (**1.8**). The diagnosis of asthma is confirmed in individuals in whom the FEV_1 or peak flow improves by more than 15%. Absence of such an improvement does not necessarily mean an individual

does not have asthma – patients may not have airflow obstruction at the time of the test, may have taken a β-agonist before the test, or may have more fixed airflow obstruction. In these individuals, the diagnosis is clarified by home peak flow monitoring. Assessment of bronchodilator responsiveness is therefore most helpful if the peak flow is low to start with, although it is worth doing in all individuals at the time the diagnosis is considered, as it will enable the maximum peak flow rate to be determined.

- *Response to exercise* is primarily used in children who are well at the time and, as a result, it may be difficult to confirm the diagnosis of asthma. The child's peak flow is recorded and then the child runs for 6 minutes with a peak flow being recorded every 10 minutes for 30 minutes after stopping. Once again a fall in peak flow of more than 15% would confirm the diagnosis of asthma (**1.9**).
- *Response to corticosteroid therapy* – in some patients with relatively fixed airflow obstruction in whom the diagnosis of asthma is still suspected, improvement in lung function (FEV_1 or peak flow) following a trial of oral or inhaled corticosteroid therapy may be useful in confirming the diagnosis (**1.7, 1.8**).

Table 1.2 Objective measurements

>20% diurnal variation on ≥3 days in a week for two weeks on peak expiratory flow diary

or FEV_1 ≥15% (and 200 ml) increase after short-acting $β_2$-agonist (e.g. salbutamol 400 µg by metered dose inhaler + spacer or 2.5 mg by nebulizer)

or FEV_1 ≥15% (and 200 ml) increase after 6-week trial of inhaled steroids or a 2-week trial of oral steroids

or FEV_1 ≥15% decrease after 6 minutes of exercise (running)

FEV_1, forced expiratory volume in 1 second.

Investigations

Chest radiography is characteristically normal in uncomplicated asthma and as a result is not undertaken in the routine diagnosis of asthma. A chest X-ray would be undertaken if another diagnosis is suspected or in patients with severe asthma for a specific reason (e.g. to assess an alternative diagnosis such as allergic bronchopulmonary aspergillosis). Measurement of non-specific bronchial responsiveness is not

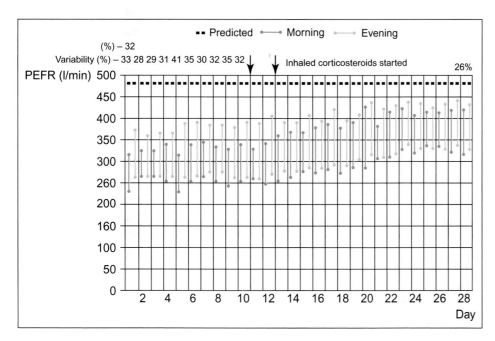

1.7 Daily peak flow records in an asthmatic subject showing variability in peak expiratory flow rate (PEFR). These records, before and after bronchodilator in the morning and evening for a month, show the effect of inhaled steroids which were introduced after 10 days. The lower bullet in each pair of readings represents the value before bronchodilator, the upper bullet the value after bronchodilator. Courtesy of ST Holgate.

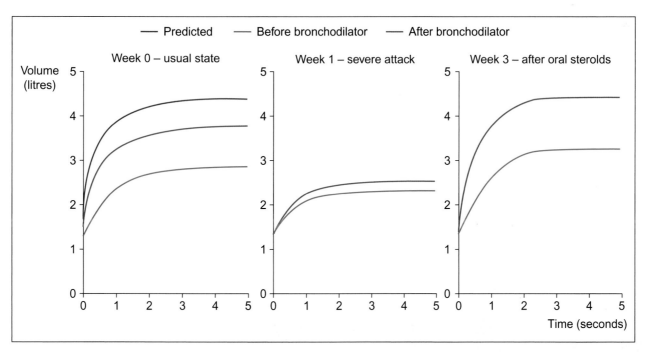

1.8 Bronchodilator responsiveness in a patient with asthma. The response of the forced expiratory volume in one second (FEV$_1$) and the forced vital capacity (FVC) to inhaled bronchodilator are shown, together with the predicted value (left). The response to bronchodilator before and after a week of treatment with oral steroids (middle and right). Courtesy of ST Holgate.

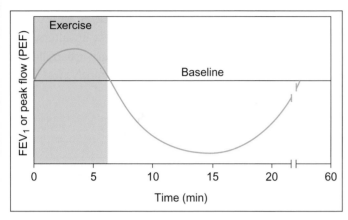

1.9 A typical asthmatic response to an exercise test, showing initial bronchodilation, followed by bronchoconstriction after 6 minutes of exercise. Courtesy of ST Holgate.

Table 1.3 Conditions that may present in a manner similar to asthma

- Chronic obstructive pulmonary disease
- Left ventricular failure
- Central airways obstruction/foreign body
- Drug use (e.g. angiotensin-converting enzyme inhibitors)
- Pulmonary embolism
- Laryngeal causes of airways obstruction including vocal cord dysfunction
- Tracheal pathology such as tumour
- Bronchiectasis
- Gastro-oesophageal reflux

recommended in the routine diagnosis of asthma because it is neither sensitive nor specific for asthma, but may be occasionally useful if the diagnosis is difficult. Although airways inflammation represents the underlying disease process in asthma, routine measurement of biological markers of airways inflammation such as sputum eosinophils, serum eosinophil cationic protein or exhaled nitric oxide is not currently recommended. However, monitoring exhaled nitric oxide, sputum eosinophils or bronchial hyper-responsiveness has shown some promise in terms of monitoring asthma control as a guide to treatment requirements.

Differential diagnosis

Asthma is quite common, so it is easy to miss other disorders that may present in a similar manner. Consideration of differential diagnoses is therefore worthwhile, depending on the presentation, as shown in *Table 1.3*[7].

These alternative diagnoses should particularly be considered in patients who do not respond as expected to a standard management regimen.

Provoking factors

Identification of provoking factors is not only helpful in terms of making the diagnosis of asthma, but this aspect of the history may also signal to the patient the underlying disease severity, for example if asthma symptoms are frequently triggered by exercise, fumes or at night-time, this is a sign of unstable asthma[6] (*Table 1.4*).

Changes in climate can trigger asthma symptoms through changes in temperature and humidity as well as other factors such as the release of allergenic pollen particles. The focus on air pollution is often on outdoor sources such as vehicle exhaust fumes, however, indoor sources such as cooking or heating with natural gas, coal or wood are also important, as are household varnishes and cleaning chemicals, particularly in those who spend most of their time indoors. Similarly, both indoor and outdoor allergens can provoke asthma symptoms. The most common allergens that people with asthma are sensitized to are house dust mite, cat and dog dander, cockroach, pollens and moulds (**1.10**).

Asthma can also be provoked by a wide range of foods, additives and preservatives, which usually can only be identified by careful monitoring. These include foods to which a person may be allergic, such as egg, peanuts and shellfish, preservatives such as tartrazine (orange colouring) and sulphites (in certain alcoholic drinks such as wine).

Occupational asthma

In making the diagnosis of asthma in adults, it is important to consider the possibility of occupational asthma, in which asthma may develop as a direct consequence of repeated exposure to substances in the workplace[8]. The key clues to recognizing occupational asthma are someone developing asthma for the first time as an adult, (or someone whose asthma gets a lot worse in adult life) and if someone experiences improvements in their asthma at weekends and holiday periods. The characteristic pattern is that asthma symptoms

Table 1.4 Stimuli that can provoke asthma symptoms

- Cold air

- Exercise

- Climate, including changes in temperature and humidity, e.g. fog

- Air pollution, both indoor and outdoor

- Fumes, including smoke, perfume, sprays

- Allergens, including house dust mite, cat, dog, moulds

- Medications, including

    - β-blockers used for heart disease and high blood pressure

    - non-steroidal anti-inflammatory drugs such as aspirin used for pain relief or arthritis

- Emotion, including stress and loss (bereavement)

- Hormonal, such as premenstrual and during pregnancy

- Night-time and early morning

- Foods, including preservatives, such as tartrazine (orange colouring), monosodium glutamate (used in Chinese food), sulphites (included in some wines) and allergens such as peanuts, shellfish

- Workplace exposure to agents to which individuals become sensitized

- Alcohol

- Viral respiratory tract infections such as the common cold and influenza

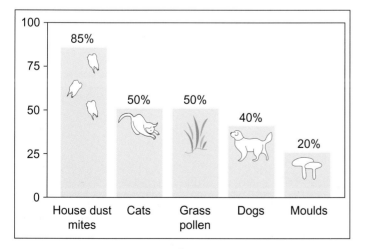

1.10 Proportions of asthmatic children sensitized to the common allergens. Courtesy of ST Holgate.

gradually develop and worsen months to years after starting a particular job. Initially the symptoms may occur only with exposure to the substance in the workplace, however with time, their asthma will occur in other situations (such as with exercise, cold air) similar to other people with asthma. Hundreds of different substances can cause occupational asthma, but the main jobs in which occupational asthma has been reported are listed in *Table 1.5*.

Confirmation of the diagnosis of occupational asthma requires a period of lung function monitoring, in which there is a characteristic pattern of a worsening of lung function at work, and improvement away from work is noted (**1.11**).

Severity

In making a diagnosis of asthma it is informative to determine the underlying severity of the disease[2, 5]. The rationale for determining severity is that treatment is based on the level of asthma control and that if the patient is classified

Table 1.5 Common occupations associated with asthma

- Spray painters
- Sawmill workers or carpenters
- Bakers
- Smelter workers
- Electronics workers
- Pharmaceutical industry workers

correctly they are more likely to receive the right treatment. In this way, people with asthma are considered to have either persistent or intermittent asthma, depending on whether their symptoms occur on most days (persistent) or only occasionally (intermittent) (*Table 1.6*). People with persistent asthma are further classified into mild, moderate and severe, depending on the level of their symptoms, lung function impairment and the amount of treatment required to control their asthma.

The high-risk asthmatic patient

A related objective in determining the underlying level of asthma severity is to identify individuals who are at consid-

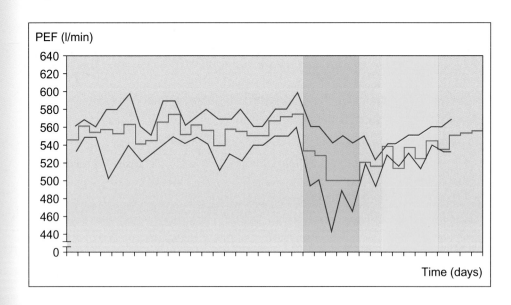

1.11 Characteristic pattern of lung function in occupational asthma: the pink shaded area represents the 5-day period back at work, and the yellow shaded area a period working at another area without exposure to the suspected agent. PEF, peak expiratory flow. Courtesy of ST Holgate.

Table 1.6 Classification of asthma severity by clinical features before starting treatment

Intermittent	• Occasional brief symptoms (<1–2 times/week during day; <1–2 times/month at night)
	• Peak flow >80% predicted and variability <20%
Persistent mild	• Symptoms (<1 time/day but ≥1–2 times/week during the day; <1 time/week but >1–2 times/month at night)
	• Peak flow >70–80% predicted and variability <20–30%
Moderate	• Daily symptoms, symptoms at night >1 time/week
	• Peak flow >60–70% predicted and variability >30%
Severe	• Daily symptoms
	• Frequent symptoms at night
	• Limitation of daily activities
	• Peak flow <60% predicted and variability >30%

erably greater risk than others in terms of a serious outcome such as a life-threatening attack[9, 10]. Such high-risk individuals can be identified by the presence of one or more risk factors which relate either to factors that negatively affect behaviour or access to medical care or to underlying past asthma severity (*Table 1.7*)[11].

Table 1.7 Identifying the high-risk asthmatic patient: markers of risk*

- Adolescents

- Disadvantaged racial groups

- Psychological or psychosocial problems

- Three or more asthma medications prescribed

- Requirement for more than two reliever or bronchodilator inhalers per month

- Frequent visits to general practitioner for unstable asthma

- One or more hospital emergency department visits in the past year

- Recent hospital admission for asthma

- Previous admission to intensive care unit or high dependency unit for asthma

* The greater the number of risk factors present, the greater the risk of a life-threatening attack

---

References

1. Fletcher CM, Gilson J, Hugh–Jones P, Scadding JG (1999). Terminology, definitions, and classification of chronic pulmonary emphysema and related conditions: a report of the conclusions of a CIBA guest symposium. *Thorax*, **14**:286–299.

2. Global Initiative for Asthma (GINA) (2005). *Global Strategy for Asthma Management and Prevention.* Bethesda: National Institutes of Health. Available online at: www.ginasthma.org (accessed 16 May 2006).

3. Djukanovic R, Roche WR, Wilson JW, Beasley CR, Twentyman OP, Howarth RH, Holgate ST (1990). Mucosal inflammation in asthma. State of the Art. *Am Rev Respir Dis*, **142**:434–457.

4. Sterk PJ, Fabbri LM, Quanjer PH, Cockcroft DW, O'Byrne PM, Anderson SD, Juniper EF, Malo JL (1993). Airway responsiveness. Standardized challenge testing with pharmacological, physical and sensitizing stimuli in adults. Report Working Party Standardization of Lung Function Tests, European Community for Steel and Coal. Official Statement of the European Respiratory Society. *Eur Resp J*, **6**(Suppl 16):53–83.

5. British Thoracic Society and Scottish Intercollegiate Guidelines Network (2003). British Guideline on Asthma Management: a national clinical guideline. *Thorax*, **58**(Suppl 1):i1–94.

6. Beasley R, Town I, Fitzharris P (2003). Diagnosis and assessment of asthma. In: *Respiratory Medicine*, Volume 2, 3rd edition. Gibson GJ, Geddes DM, Costabel U, Sterk PJ, Corrin B (eds). Elsevier Science, Edinburgh pp. 1306–1322.

7. Grammar LC, Greenberger PA (1992). Diagnosis and classification of asthma. *Chest* **101**(Suppl):S393–395.

8. Chan-Yeung M, Malo J-L (2000). Epidemiology of occupational asthma. In: *Asthma and Rhinitis*, 2nd edition. Busse WW, Holgate ST (eds). Blackwell Scientific, Oxford, pp 43–55.

9. Nelson HS (2000). Recalcitrant asthma. In: *Asthma and Rhinitis*, 2nd edition. Busse WW, Holgate ST (eds). Blackwell Scientific, Oxford, pp 1864–1879.

10. American Thoracic Society (2000). Proceedings of the ATS Workshop on Refractory Asthma: current understanding, recommendations and unanswered questions. *Am J Respir Crit Care Med*, **162**:2341–2351.

11. Miles J, Fitzharris P, Beasley R (1995). An approach to the management of the 'high risk' asthmatic. *Clin Immunother*, **4**(6):445–450.

Further reading

Holgate ST, Boushey HA, Fabbri LM (eds) (1999). *Difficult Asthma*. Martin Dunitz, London.

O'Byrne PM, Thomson NC (eds) (2001). *Manual of Asthma Management*, 2nd edition. WB Saunders, London.

Chapter 2

Epidemiology of Asthma

Peter Burney

Definition of asthma

The lack of a definition for asthma (see **Chapter 1**) is important, particularly for epidemiologists. For lack of a true definition against which it would be possible to evaluate an instrument to assess whether someone has asthma, it is necessary to use pragmatic definitions that are not verifiable as 'valid' instruments. Several of these have been suggested (*Table 2.1*) although none is entirely satisfactory. In the USA the practice of asking about 'doctor diagnosed' asthma has been popular as a way of identifying people with asthma and this has the advantages both of simplicity and of eliciting highly repeatable answers. It is also the case that the asthmatic patients identified in this way are rarely judged by any other methods as not being asthmatic. The disadvantages are that this fails to identify undiagnosed cases and this may be a serious problem, particularly for instance when assessing the response of health services. It also has a disadvantage in international surveys where, at least in the past, the use of diagnostic terms appears to have differed significantly between countries[4].

An alternative strategy is to devise a questionnaire to elicit the typical symptoms of asthma. This has the advantage of making explicit the criteria by which someone is labelled and avoids the necessity of relying on what is likely to be a very variable process to reach a decision on whether someone has the condition. However, there is no symptom list that is likely to be entirely sufficient to make a clear distinction between asthma and other conditions affecting the airway. It is also still dependent on the perception and recognition of these symptoms by the individual affected, and this is also likely to be very variable.

The third general method that has been used is to take some physiological measure believed to be characteristic

Table 2.1 Pragmatic definitions of asthma
A doctor's diagnosis
Symptoms
• Wheeze accompanied by shortness of breath
• Waking at night with breathlessness
Airway responsiveness in response to
• Histamine, methacholine
• Adenosine, hypertonic solutions
• Exercise, cold dry air

of the disease, in this case generally a measure of airway hyper-responsiveness. For large surveys this is a more costly procedure and for the measures used most often, response to histamine or methacholine, is again not entirely specific for asthma, those with other airways disease such as chronic obstructive pulmonary disease also responding positively to the tests. The method is, however, independent of perception on the part of the subjects.

Geographical variation

Although there is no 'validated' method of diagnosing asthma, it is still possible to draw conclusions about the disease provided that well-standardized methods are used, and in epidemiological studies standardization is extremely important. Data can only be validly compared if they are collected using similar and therefore comparable methods. Whichever method is used to collect information on the prevalence of asthma, large variations in prevalence have been reported. They do not necessarily provide similar results, however, if different methods are used (**2.1, 2.2** show the distribution of diagnosed asthma and of measured airway responsiveness as measured in the European Community Respiratory Health Survey [ECRHS]). Diagnosed asthma is notably high (significantly above the median prevalence) in almost all the English-speaking countries, and in Sweden, whereas airway responsiveness is significantly below the median rate for the study, for instance, in three of the six Canadian centres and two of the three Swedish centres.

Time trends

To understand the time trends for asthma, studies are needed that measure the prevalence of disease using standardized methods in the same populations at different time points. There are now many such studies. The upward trend in asthma prevalence from the middle of the twentieth century to the mid-1990s is seen in **2.3**. Only since that time have a few studies started to show a slowing down of the increase or a reverse in the trend. The prevalence

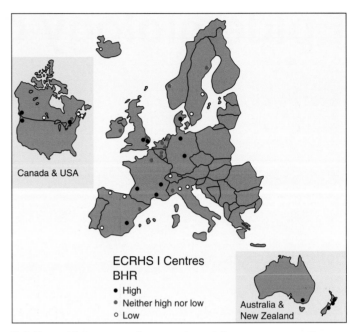

2.2 Bronchial responsiveness is not the same as asthma but most people with asthma do have increased bronchial reactivity Some people who do not have asthma, particularly older smokers and those with atopy, will also demonstrate some bronchial reactivity. In this map, centres with high levels of bronchial responsiveness using a standardized protocol are shown in black and low level areas are shown in white. As can be seen, centres in Australia and New Zealand, two centres in England and three centres in Canada have high levels of bronchial responsiveness and have already reported high levels of asthma. The southern part of Europe (Galdakao) – Italy and some centres in Spain – have low bronchial reactivity. In Iceland there is low bronchial reactivity. In general the geographical distribution of bronchial reactivity is similar to that seen for asthma prevalence BUT this is not always the case, for example Sweden had a high prevalence of reported asthma but does not have a high prevalence of bronchial reactivity.

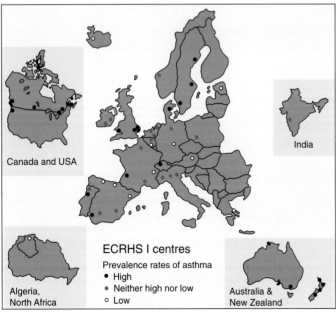

2.1 This map shows the prevalence of asthma as defined by the reporting of 'having an asthma attack in the last 12 months OR the current use of asthma medication'. Centres that are marked with a red dot are those with a high prevalence and those with a green dot have a low prevalence.

of disease is shown on a logarithmic scale which displays similar percentage increases from different starting points as parallel. The overall variation in prevalence is seen to be very variable and this reflects both differences in methods (studies of wheeze giving much higher estimates of prevalence than studies of diagnosed asthma) and differences in underlying prevalence in different locations. However, from the middle of the 1950s to the 1990s there is an almost universal upward trend which represents a doubling of the

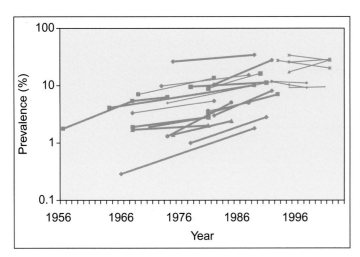

2.3 Changing prevalence of asthma and wheeze.

prevalence approximately every 15 years. This appears to reflect an increase in the prevalence of people who have a measurable immunoglobulin ε (IgE) to specific allergens (**2.4**). Although these studies are much rarer, they seem to confirm that what is being observed in the studies based on questionnaires is likely to be real, rather than simply a tendency to report more in questionnaires.

Similar indirect evidence for a real increase came much earlier from an analysis of admissions data for England[5]. The increase in male admissions to English hospitals attributed to asthma from the 1950s to the 1980s is shown in **2.5**. Again the admission rates are plotted on a logarithmic scale.

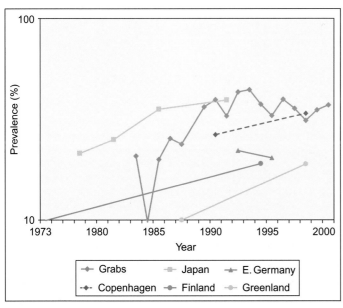

2.4 Changing prevalence of specific IgE to common allergens.

The admission rates for children increased ten-fold over this period, and there was a slower increase among older age groups. This has generally been interpreted as demonstrating that this problem is a paediatric problem, and it has been argued whether this is likely to reflect a change in prevalence or a change in medical practice, with a greater likelihood of children being admitted. The same data are re-plotted in **2.6** by the year of birth of the patients, rather than by the date of admission. This suggests that this is not strictly an age-related phenomenon. The simpler explanation is that it is related to when people were born. This so-called 'birth cohort effect' is less likely to be due to changes in medical practice which would be expected to affect all ages at the same time, and possibly more likely to be due to a change in prevalence of disease determined by events in early life. A similar plot for girls and women (**2.7**) shows a similar effect with an upward displacement of rates for women in their child-bearing years, reflecting other observations suggesting that these women have a higher prevalence of asthma.

This birth cohort effect has also been shown for sensitization to allergens. The prevalence of sensitization to common allergens in the first ECRHS is shown in **2.8**. Sensitization was measured as positive identification of IgE against mite, grass, cat or *Cladosporium*. It shows a lower prevalence of sensitization in the older age groups and this pattern has been previously noted and generally interpreted as a change in sensitization with age. However, the results of a follow-up study strongly suggest that this is an unlikely explanation[6] (**2.9**). There is no reduction in prevalence of sensitization among individuals almost 10 years later, suggesting strongly that the apparent age effect is in fact a 'birth cohort effect'. The implication of this for the future of the current epidemic of atopic disease is important. Some of the most recent studies in children, particularly in more affluent countries, suggest that the current epidemic is now abating. If the current epidemic is related to a birth cohort effect it will take many years for this change to work into the older population which is most affected by asthma and its complications.

The causes of the epidemic

It has been surprisingly difficult to provide clear and direct evidence to explain the increase in sensitization and asthma. This is in part because the evidence has not been collected in the right historical cohorts. Exceptions to this are the British national birth cohorts of 1958 and 1970. In these cohorts

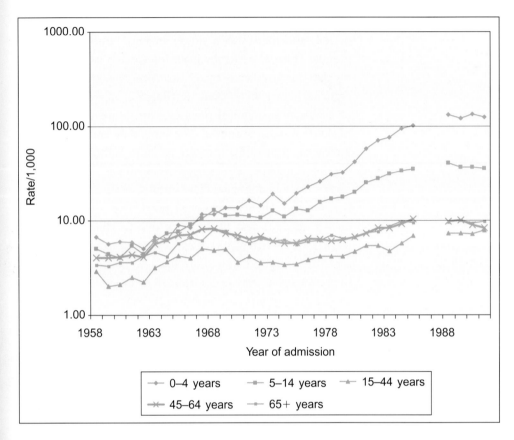

2.5 Male asthma admissions by year of admission.

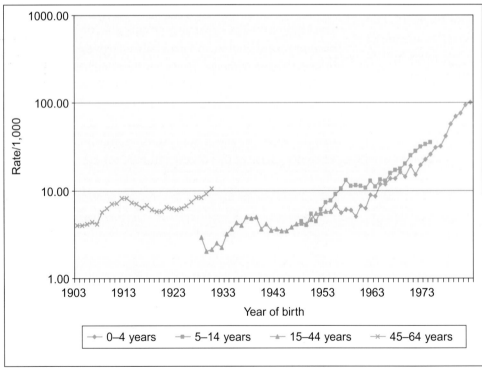

2.6 Male asthma admissions by year of birth.

information on at least some of the potential risk factors was collected. However none of them appeared to explain the increase in reported prevalence of wheezy illness[7]. *Table 2.2* shows the odds ratio for asthma/wheezy bronchitis at age 16 years in the 1970 cohort compared with the same condition at the same age in the 1958 cohort both before and after

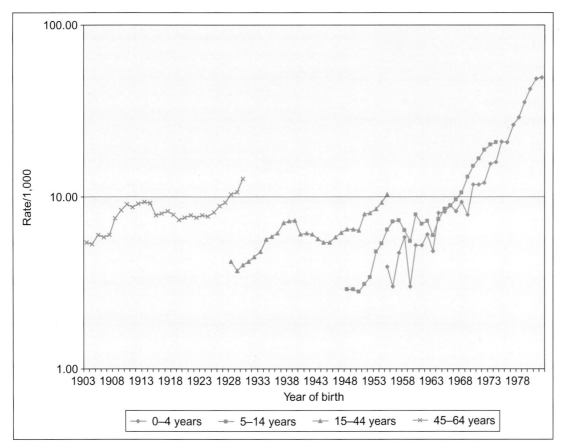

2.7 Female asthma admissions by year of birth.

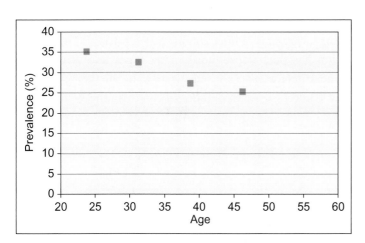

2.8 Prevalence of sensitization in ECRHS I.

adjusting for specific risk factors. Small differences in the unadjusted ratios are due to slight differences in the individuals who could be included in the analyses. If any of the risk factors could explain part of the increase between the cohorts, the adjusted odds ratio would have been substantially lower than the unadjusted odds ratio. It can be clearly seen that none of the odds ratios changed substantially on adjustment.

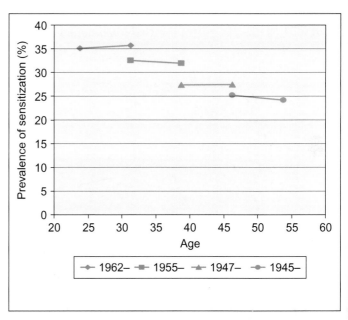

2.9 Longitudinal changes in sensitization (any allergen) by birth cohort.

Table 2.2 Changes in prevalence of asthma/wheezy bronchitis in 16-year-olds from 1974 to 1986 before and after adjustment for potential risk factors

Risk factor	Unadjusted odds ratio	Adjusted odds ratio
Birthweight	1.77	1.77
Maternal age	1.75	1.71
Breastfeeding	1.80	1.78
Birth order	1.72	1.72
Maternal age	1.72	1.70
Child's smoking	1.79	1.82
Father's social class	1.71	1.71
Sex	1.76	1.77

Table 2.3 shows a similar analysis from the National Study of Health and Growth investigating the possible effect of changes in body mass index (BMI)[8]. There are many studies now that have shown some association between reported asthma and asthma-like symptoms and high BMI, particularly among women. It is also known that BMI and asthma have been increasing markedly in many countries over the past few decades. The possibility that the trend in BMI could explain the increase in asthma was a serious one. However, the results of this analysis of a mixed longitudinal study of English and Scottish primary school children shows that the one trend cannot explain the other and further study showed that the time trends although similar did not coincide in detail.

BMI is determined by both diet and energy expenditure. Other aspects of diet have also been implicated in determining the prevalence of asthma. Most prominently, the amount of antioxidant in the diet has been suggested as an important determinant, and there is some evidence that some antioxidants have declined at least in the British diet over the past few decades[9]. Several cross-sectional studies have shown an inverse relation between intake of various potential antioxidants such as selenium (*Table 2.4*) and apples (*Table 2.5*) and asthma[10]. So far, however, there is no direct evidence that lack of antioxidants has been the cause of the increase in asthma and there is little direct experimental evidence for a causative relation between antioxidant intake and the prevalence of asthma. The evidence for protection against exacerbations induced by oxidant stress is, however, stronger.

The 'hygiene hypothesis'

In 1989 the observation was made that hay fever (though not asthma) was less common in those from large families, and the hypothesis was put forward that this might be because of the lower rates of infection in small sibships[11]. This observation has been reproduced many times and also shown to be true for rates of sensitization to allergens (**2.10**)[12]. The theoretical underpinning of this hypothesis has come

Table 2.3 Changing prevalence of asthma and wheeze in UK boys aged 8–9 years, 1982–1994

	Relative risk/year (95% confidence interval)	
	Unadjusted trend	Trend adjusted for BMI
Asthma attack	1.08	1.08
	(1.06 to 1.10)	(1.06 to1.10)
Wheeze	1.04	1.03
	(1.02 to 1.05)	(1.02 to 1.05)
Attack of asthma or bronchitis	1.04	1.04
	(1.02 to 1.06)	(1.02 to 1.06)

Table 2.4 Antioxidant trace elements and asthma: selenium[9]

Intake/day (quintiles)	Odds ratio*	95% confidence interval
1	1.0	
2	0.95	0.66 to 1.36
3	0.69	0.46 to 1.03
4	0.53	0.34 to 0.81
5	0.56	0.35 to 0.89

*Adjusted odds ratio *P* trend 0.0015.

Table 2.5 Flavonoid-rich foods and asthma: apples[9]

Intake	Odds ratio*	95% confidence interval
<Once/month	1.0	
1–3 ×/month	0.96	0.69 to 1.34
Once/week	0.90	0.63 to 1.30
2–4 ×/week	0.68	0.48 to 0.95
≥5 ×/week	0.68	0.47 to 0.98

*Adjusted odds ratio *P* trend 0.0057.

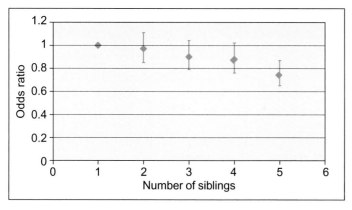

2.10 Association between family size and prevalence of atopy (radioallergosorbent test [RAST] +). Redrawn from Svanes C *et al.* (1999). Childhood environment and adult atopy: Results from the European Community Respiratory Health Survey (1999). *J Allergy Clin Immunol,* **103**:415–420.

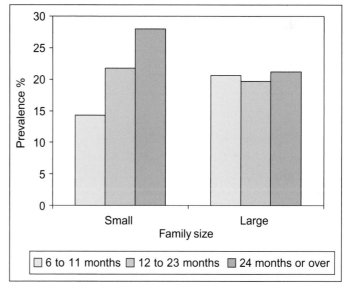

2.11 Effect of family size and age at going to school on prevalence of positive skin prick tests in later life. Redrawn from Kramer *et al.* (1999). Age of entry to day nursery and allergy in later childhood. *Lancet,* **353**:450–454.

from a number of sources. First, there is evidence, mostly from mice, that the immune system can be polarized to respond with a non-allergic type of response (T helper [Th]1 response) by early exposure to infections. Second, it has been shown that for those from small families early exposure to other children in daycare settings can act in the same way to protect from allergic types of response (**2.11**)[13]. Finally it has been shown that the risk of allergy is inversely related to serological evidence of enteric infections (though not of other childhood infections) (**2.12**)[14]. This general hypothesis has been used also to explain the protective effect of being brought up on a farm (**2.13**)[15]. The principal

objection to this hypothesis as explained by an imbalance of Th1/Th2 responses is that there seems to be no reciprocal relation between responses in the same organ relating to Th1 and Th2 responses. For instance, first, there is no inverse association between atopic eczema and psoriasis. Second, under the initial hypothesis it might be expected that as atopic (Th2) diseases increased, there would be a fall in Th1-related diseases such as diabetes mellitus, and this has clearly not been the case.

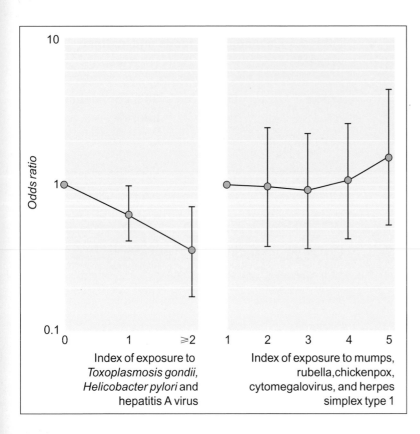

2.12 Relation between infection and risk of allergy. Reproduced from Matricardi PM *et al.* (2000). Cross-sectional retrospective study of prevalence of atopy among Italian military students with antibodies against hepatitis A virus. *Br Med J*, **320**: 412–417.

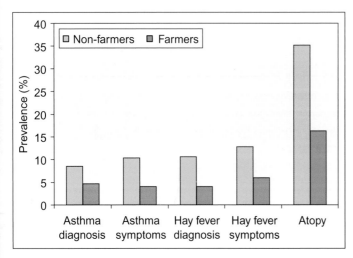

2.13 Effect of a farming environment on allergic disease in children participating in the ALEX study. From Riedler *et al.* (2001). Exposure to farming in early life and development of asthma and allergy: a cross-sectional survey. *Lancet*, **358**(9288):1129–1433.

The developing world

As has been pointed out, there is relatively little chance of using historical data to test hypotheses relating to the causes of the epidemic, as the data needed have not usually been collected. There is a much better chance looking at contemporary differences between high and low prevalence areas. The most stark differences in this regard have been found between the urban and rural areas of less developed countries. A number of early surveys showed stark differences in prevalence and are shown in **2.14**, again foreshortened by a logarithmic scale[16–19]. The results of these studies were mostly based on questionnaire data but have been confirmed by exercise tests as demonstrated by studies from Zimbabwe (**2.15**)[20]. In these studies there was a progressive increase in the prevalence of exercise-induced bronchospasm from the remote rural area (Wedza) to the poor urban area (South Harare) to the affluent suburb of North Harare. In the affluent suburb there was no difference in prevalence between the white and black children, strongly suggesting that this difference is related to the environment.

From what has been said above about the hygiene hypothesis and an early observation from Guinea–Bissau that

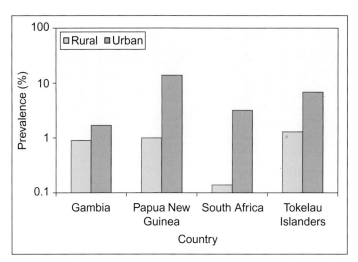

2.14 Early studies of urban–rural differences in the prevalence of asthma.

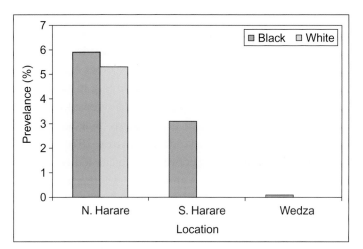

2.15 Prevalence of exercise-induced bronchoconstriction in three areas of Zimbabwe. From Keeley DJ, Gallivan S (1991). Comparison of the prevalence of reversible airways obstruction in rural and urban Zimbabwean children. *Thorax*, **468**:549–553.

children from families who kept pigs had a lower prevalence of sensitization[21], it might be supposed that the hygiene hypothesis would be a good explanation for the findings in the developing world. This is, however, not likely to be the case. Earlier studies from Zimbabwe show clearly that there is no lack of sensitization in the rural areas, indeed grass sensitization is much higher in rural areas among those with no asthma than it is in asthmatic patients in the urban areas (**2.16**)[22]. Similar observations have been made elsewhere and what is different in these rural areas is not a failure to sensitize against allergens, but a failure to develop skin responses

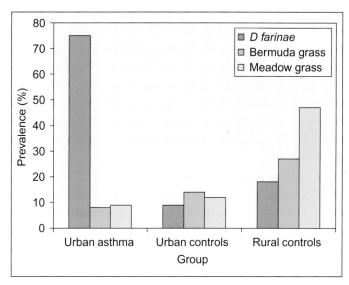

2.16 Specific IgE to inhalant allergens in two areas of Zimbabwe.

to the allergens (**2.17**)[23]. Exercise-induced bronchoconstriction is also unlinked to evidence of sensitization in the rural areas (**2.18**).

A separate explanation has been put forward for this in terms of the balance not of Th1 and Th2 responses but of Th and T regulatory (Treg) cells. This hypothesizes that some poorly pathogenic infections or infestations, including parasitic infestations, elicit a strong regulatory response that

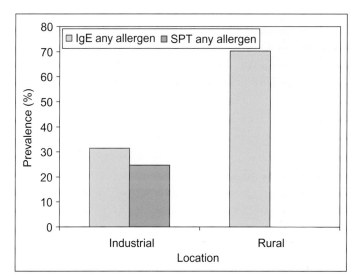

2.17 Prevalence of sensitization among primary school-children in two locations in Kenya using specific IgE and skin prick tests (SPT). Adapted from Perzanowski MS *et al.* (2001). Atopy, asthma, and antibodies to Ascaris among rural and urban children in Kenya. *J Pediatr*, **140**:582–588.

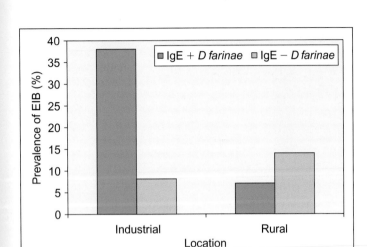

2.18 Prevalence of exercise-induced bronchoconstriction (EIB) among Kenyan schoolchildren in two areas according to sensitization measured by specific IgE. Adapted from Perzanowski MS *et al.* (2001). Atopy, asthma, and antibodies to Ascaris among rural and urban children in Kenya. *J Pediatr*, **140**:582–588.

damps down inflammatory responses. Some evidence of this has been provided by a study of the influence of schistosome infestations on skin test responses to mites (**2.19**)[24]. At the back of this diagram a clear relation is seen between the skin test response to mite and the presence of mite-specific IgE, as would be expected. However, this relation is attenuated as the interleukin (IL)-10 response to schistosome antigen increases. IL-10 is a cytokine strongly associated with Treg responses. Although these findings are sometimes discussed as if they are in some sense equivalent to the original hygiene hypothesis, this is not the case. The original hypothesis was successful in explaining differences in hay fever, initially, and in sensitization rates. The Treg mechanism cannot explain these findings just as the Th1/Th2 balance cannot explain the findings in Africa.

Mortality

Mortality from asthma is clearly an important public health measure, but mortality is difficult to interpret where the prevalence rates are changing. Mortality is determined by the underlying prevalence of disease, and more specifically of severe disease, and by the fatality rate in cases. It is the fatality rate that most concerns doctors as this could be interpreted as a measure of the quality of the health services.

The reported mortality from asthma across the twentieth century is shown in **2.20**[25]. Rates in the older age groups are difficult to interpret as at all these periods the relative prevalence of asthma and other obstructive lung diseases would have been very small and the rates would have been strongly influenced by misclassification. It is not unreasonable to suppose that the decline in asthma mortality is a reflection of the declining mortality rates from chronic obstructive pulmonary disease.

For the younger age group there appears to have been more evidence for an increase over this period of time (particularly for the 15–24-year-olds). This may reflect an increasing prevalence of disease. Superimposed on these trends there are periodic increases in mortality. That seen during World War I, most markedly in 25–34-year-olds, probably reflects the loss of fit men without asthma to the military services (who are not included in the statistics). The short-lived increase at the beginning of World War II and seen in all age groups is thought to represent the effects of a respiratory epidemic. More marked than either of these was the epidemic most obvious among the young in the 1960s. This was examined at the time and attributed to the wide availability and over-reliance on the early β-agonist inhalers. The resurgence of these deaths in the 1970s following the introduction of selective β$_2$-agonists led to further investigation of these deaths and debate whether the deaths were associated with continuing over-reliance on β-agonists and under-use of inhaled steroids, or to the introduction of stronger β-agonists with allegedly less broncho-specific action[26,27].

Conclusions

There is early evidence that in some of the richer countries, at least, the relentless increase in the prevalence of asthma seen over the second half of the twentieth century has begun to recede. However, this is not yet seen in other countries and the current evidence is that the epidemic will not be reversed in those birth cohorts already affected. In other words, the epidemic is likely to cast a long shadow forward and is still to have its most profound effects in poorer countries. This has three consequences for policy-based research. The first is that there are still requirements for understanding how best to effectively manage the risks posed to allergic people, both in the home and at work, and to develop better secondary

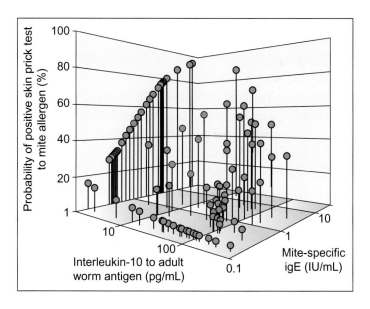

2.19 Probability of a positive skin reaction to mite allergens for given concentrations of mite-specific IgE (IU/mL) and interleukin-10 to adult worm antigen (pg/mL). Reproduced from van den Biggelaar AHJ *et al.* (2000). Decreased atopy in children infected with *Schistosoma haematobium*: a role for parasite-induced interleukin-10. *Lancet*, **356**:1723–1727.

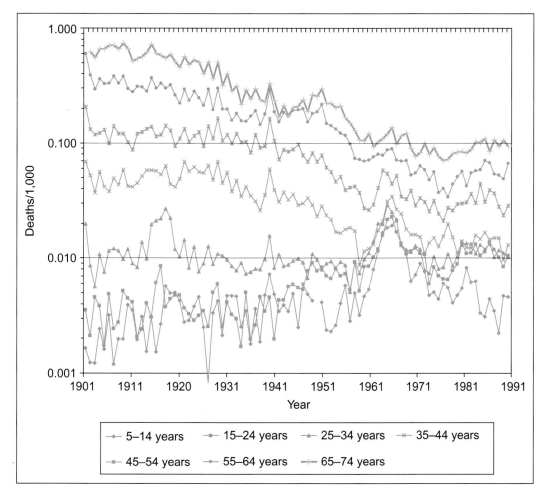

2.20 Male asthma mortality: England and Wales.

prevention for these people. Secondly, there is a need to improve the management of the disease in those who have developed it. Finally, there is still a need to understand the origins of the epidemic which is still a problem in poorer countries with relatively few resources to cope with the problem.

References

1. Fletcher CM, Gilson J, Hugh-Jones P, Scadding JG (1999). Terminology, definitions, and classification of chronic pulmonary emphysema and related conditions: a report of the conclusions of a CIBA guest symposium. *Thorax*, **14**:286–299.

2. Scadding JG (1963). Meaning of diagnostic terms in broncho-pulmonary disease. *Br Med J*, **2**:1425–1430.

3. National Heart, Lung, and Blood Institute, National Institutes of Health (1992). International consensus report on diagnosis and treatment of asthma. National Heart, Lung, and Blood Institute, National Institutes of Health, Bethesda, Maryland 20892. Publication no. 92-3091, March.

4. Burney P (1989). The effect of death certification practice on recorded national asthma mortality rates. *Rev Epidemiol Sante Publique*, **37**:385–389.

5. Alderson M (1987). Trends in morbidity and mortality from asthma. *Popul Trends*, **49**:18–23.

6. Jarvis D, Luczynska C, Chinn S, Potts J, Sunyer J, Janson C, Svanes C, Kunzli N, Leynaert B, Heinrich J, Kerkhof M, Ackermann-Liebrich U, Anto JM, Cerveri I, de Marco R, Gislason T, Neukirch F, Vermeire P, Wjst M, Burney P (2005). Change in prevalence of IgE sensitization and mean total IgE with age and cohort. *J Allergy Clin Immunol*, **116**:675–682.

7. Lewis S, Butland B, Strachan D, Bynner J, Richards D, Butler N, Britton J (1996). Study of the aetiology of wheezing illness at age 16 in two national British birth cohorts. *Thorax*, **517**:670–676.

8. Chinn S, Rona RJ (2001). Can the increase in body mass index explain the rising trend in asthma in children. *Thorax*, **56**:845–850.

9. Seaton A, Godden DJ, Brown K (1994). Increase in asthma: a more toxic environment or a more susceptible population? *Thorax*, **492**:171–174.

10. Shaheen SO, Sterne JAC, Thompson RL, Songhurst CE, Margetts BM, Burney PGJ (2002). Dietary antioxidants and asthma in adults: population based case-control study. *Am J Respir Crit Care Med*, **164**:1823–1828.

11. Strachan DP (1989). Hay fever, hygiene and household size. *Br Med J*, **299**(6710):1259–1260.

12. Svanes C, Jarvis D, Chinn S, Burney P (1999). Childhood environment and adult atopy: Results from the European Community Respiratory Health Survey. *J Allergy Clin Immunol*, **103**:415–420.

13. Kramer U, Heinrich J, Wjst M, Wichmann H-E (1999). Age of entry to day nursery and allergy in later childhood. *Lancet*, **353**:450–454.

14. Matricardi PM, Rosmini F, Ferrigno L, Nisini R, Rapicetta M, Chionne P, Stroffolini T, Pasquini P, D'Amelio R (1997). Cross sectional retrospective study of prevalence of atopy among Italian military students with antibodies against hepatitis A virus. *Br Med J*, **314**:999–1003.

15. Riedler J, Eder W, Oberfeld G, Schreuer M (2000). Austrian children living on a farm have less hay fever, asthma and allergic sensitization. *Clin Exp Allergy*, **302**:194–200.

16. Godfrey RC (1975). Asthma and IgE levels in rural and urban communities of The Gambia. *Clin Allergy*, **5**:201–207.

17. Anderson HR (1978). Respiratory abnormalities in Papua New Guinea children: the effects of locality and domestic wood smoke pollution. *Int J Epidemiol*, **7**:63–71.

18. Van Niekerk CH, Weinberg EG, Shore SC, Heese H, Van Schalkwyk J (1979). Prevalence of asthma: a comparative study of urban and rural Xhosa children. *Clin Allergy*, **9**:319–324.

19. Waite DA, Eyles EF, Tonkin SL, O'Donnell TV (1980). Asthma prevalence in Tokeluan children in two environments. *Clin Allergy*, **10**:71–75.

20. Keeley DJ, Gallivan S (1991). Comparison of the prevalence of reversible airways obstruction in rural and urban Zimbabwean children. *Thorax*, **468**:549–553.

21. Shaheen SO, Aaby P, Hall AJ, Barker DJ, Heyes CB, Shiell AW, Goudiaby A (1996). Measles and atopy in Guinea-Bissau. *Lancet*, **347**:1792–1796.

22. Merret TG, Merrett J, Cookson JB (1976). Allergy and parasites: the measurement of total and specific IgE levels in urban and rural communities in Rhodesia. *Clin Allergy*, **62**:131–134.

23. Perzanowski MS, Ng'ang'a LW, Carter MC, Odhiambo

J, Ngari P, Vaughan JW, Chapman MD, Kennedy MW, Platts-Mills TA (2002). Atopy, asthma, and antibodies to Ascaris among rural and urban children in Kenya. *J Pediatr*, **140**:582–588.

24. van den Biggelaar AH, van Ree R, Rodrigues LC, Lell B, Deelder AM, Kremsner PG, Yazdanbakhsh M (2000). Decreased atopy in children infected with Schistosoma haematobium: a role for parasite-induced interleukin-10. *Lancet*, **356**:1723–1727.

25. Marks G, Burney P (1998). Diseases of the respiratory system. In: *The Health of Adult Britain 1841–1991*. Charlton J, Murphy M (eds). Her Majesty's Stationery Office, London.

26. Crane J, Pearce N, Flatt A, Burgess C, Jackson R, Kwong T, Ball M, Beasley R (1989). Prescribed fenoterol and death from asthma in New Zealand, 1981–83: case-control study. *Lancet*, **i**:917–923.

27. Spitzer WO, Suissa S, Ernst P, Horwitz RI, Habbick B, Cockcroft D, Boivin JF, McNutt M, Buist AS, Rebuck AS (1992). The use of beta-agonists and the risk of death and near fatal death from asthma. *N Engl J Med*, **326**:501–506.

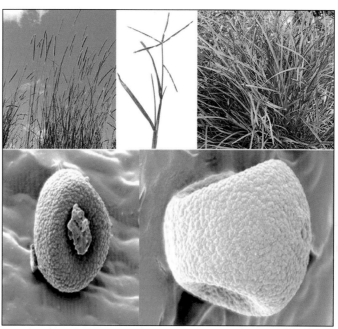

Chapter 3

Clinical Types of Asthma

Chris J Corrigan

Introduction

The rationale for identifying clinical types of asthma is to recognize facets of the disease specific for particular patients, which will have implications for clinical management and, hopefully, understanding of the precise aetiology and pathogenesis of the disease.

Atopic asthma

Atopy is defined as the propensity of certain individuals to mount an IgE response to allergens encountered at the skin and mucosal surfaces principally of the respiratory and alimentary tracts[1]. Most outdoor allergens are proteins in tree, grass and some weed pollens. Grass pollen allergy is most common (**3.1**). The season is from late May until the beginning of August. The second most important pollen is birch. Birch trees 'flower' during April and May. Proteins in birch pollen cross-react with similar proteins in other members of the birch family including alder and hazel, which flower earlier, and hornbeam, which flowers later. The main weed allergenic pollens in the UK include nettle, plantain, dock and goosefoot (**3.2**). The peak pollen season for weeds is in late summer and early autumn (**3.3**). Fungal spores which may cause allergy are ubiquitous and local concentrations vary with season, vegetation, land use and weather. The most important are *Cladosporium, Alternaria, Aspergillus* and *Penicillium* (**3.4**). Local weather conditions such as thunderstorms and pollution can cause increased allergen release[2].

The commonest source of indoor allergen is the house dust mite (see **4.9(A)**). Gut enzymes and other proteins present in the faeces are powerful allergens. House dust mites thrive in poorly ventilated, warm and humid atmospheres.

3.1 Typical allergenic grasses and some examples of their pollen. Photo courtesy of Pete Smith.

They may be responsible for allergic exacerbation of asthma, as well as rhinitis and eczema throughout the year. Domestic pets (see **4.9(D)**) and laboratory animals are the second most important source of indoor allergens in the UK. Allergenic proteins from the gut, urine or skin of these animals become trapped in airborne dander (**3.5**). Many such allergens are transported out of homes, for example stuck to clothing. The only way to reduce exposure to pets at home is not to have one, although even after removal of the pet it may take many months for the allergen reservoir to diminish. Fungal and other spores may be a significant source of allergens in the home, especially where there are damp conditions.

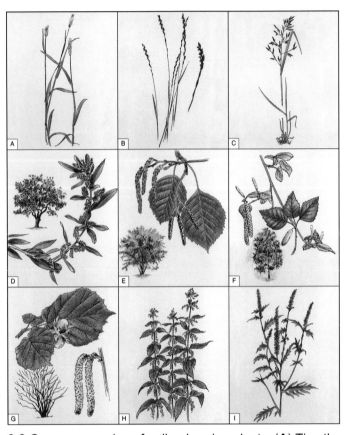

3.2 Common species of pollen-bearing plants: (**A**) Timothy grass (*Phleum pratense*); (**B**) Rye grass (*Lolium perenne*); (**C**) Meadow fescue (*Festuca pratensis*); (**D**) Olive (*Olea europaea*) (not seen in the UK); (**E**) Alder (*Alnus incana*); (**F**) Silver birch (*Betula pendula* or *verrucosa*); (**G**) Hazel (*Corylus avellana*); (**H**) Common nettle (*Urtica dioica*); (**I**) Common ragweed (*Ambrosia artemisiifolia*) (uncommon in the UK).

Food allergies arise from inappropriate IgE responses to protein allergens in foods when these enter the gut after being eaten (**3.6**). Food allergy is an important cause of exacerbation of asthma in infants and young children, although the role of food allergies in regulating asthma severity and natural history in adults is much less prominent.

Production of IgE to various allergens is readily detectable by skin prick testing (**3.7**). Dilute solutions of allergen extracts are placed on the skin then injected slightly into the surface using a sterile metal lancet. If the patient has IgE antibodies against a particular allergen, local mast cell degranulation causes a wheal reaction within 10–15 minutes of the skin prick. An alternative is to detect allergen-specific IgE in the serum, but this method is generally less sensitive (as well as more time consuming and expensive). Since many patients with allergen-specific IgE (inexplicably) show no clinical response to exposure to the allergen, clinically relevant reactions to allergens cannot be predicted from results of skin prick tests or blood tests alone. A careful history suggesting exacerbation of symptoms on exposure to the particular allergen, backed up by a positive skin prick test or blood test implicates the allergen in exacerbating disease.

Exposure to aeroallergens clearly exacerbates asthma (**3.8**) and increases the risk of acute exacerbations in allergic individuals, especially children[3]. Avoidance will improve quality of life and may reduce the need for medication. Severe allergic reactions, for example to food allergens may be potentially fatal in people with asthma. It is vital, there-

Taxa	January	February	March	April	May	June	July	August	September
Hazel (*Corylus*)									
Yew (*Taxus*)									
Alder (*Alnus*)									
Alm (*Ulmus*)									
Willow (*Salix*)									
Poplar (*Populus*)									
Birch (*Betula*)									
Ash (*Fraxinus*)									
Plane (*Plantanus*)									
Oak (*Quercus*)									
Oil seed rape (*B. napus*)									
Pine (*Pinus*)									
Grass (*Gramineae*)									
Plantain (*Plantago*)									
Lime (*Tilia*)									
Nettle (*Urtica*)									
Dock (*Rumex*)									
Mugwort (*Artemisa*)									

— Main period of pollen release
— Peak periods

3.3 Pollen calendar for the UK. Data adapted from the National Pollen and Aerobiology Research Unit, University College Worcester, Worcester, UK.

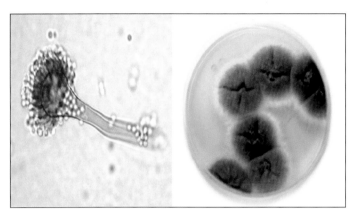

3.4 The common mould *Aspergillus fumigatus*. Common moulds are ubiquitous and their spores, produced by hyphae (see left side of picture), are allergenic. Outdoor fungi tend to sporulate in early autumn, or at other times depending on weather conditions. Fungi growing indoors in the damp may sporulate at any time.

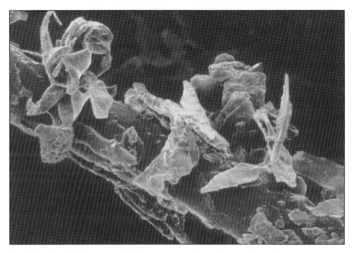

3.5 Animal dander. With permission from the American Academy of Allergy, Asthma and Immunology (www.aaaai.org).

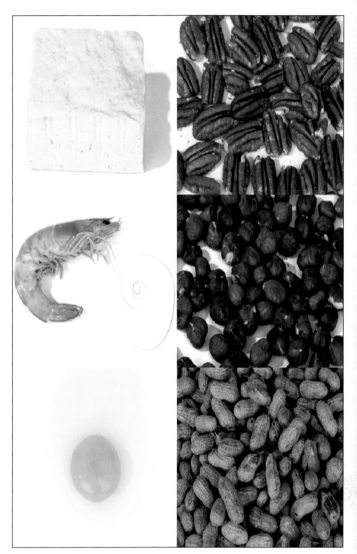

3.6 Common allergenic foods. In infants, milk and egg allergy are common in atopic children, especially with eczema. These allergies are usually transient. Later, allergies to foods such as fish, nuts and grains may appear when the child first starts to eat them. These allergies are more likely to persist. Food allergies are an important potential cause of exacerbation of asthma, rhinitis and eczema in infants and children, but less so in adults. Photo courtesy of Pete Smith.

fore, not to miss allergen triggers for asthma especially in children and adolescents. House dust mite allergy may be an important trigger in perennial asthma. Asthmatic symptoms related to animal dander are easily identified. Tree or grass pollen allergy may cause seasonal exacerbation in the spring/summer, whereas allergy to the moulds *Alternaria* or *Cladosporium* may be an important cause of severe seasonal asthma in the late summer or autumn, or perennial asthma in damp or mouldy homes. Atopic patients often have concomitant allergic rhinitis (**3.9**), which should be managed with allergen avoidance, antihistamine and topical nasal

steroid. Adequate management of rhinitis improves asthma control and reduces exacerbations. Eczema (**3.10**) is another common manifestation of the atopic diathesis and should raise the possibility of concomitant rhinitis and food allergy.

Notwithstanding the common sense of removing asthmatic patients from allergenic triggers, it has been difficult

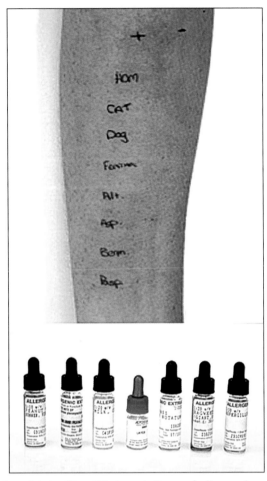

3.7 Skin prick testing. Dilute solutions of allergenic extracts are placed onto the skin and then pricked underneath the surface with a sterile metal lancet. If specific IgE is present, the resulting degranulation of local mast cells causes a wheal reaction within 10–15 minutes. Prick tests with fresh food, where possible, are preferable to extracts for the diagnosis of food allergy.

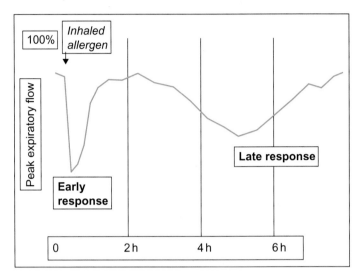

3.8 Experimental exposure of allergic asthmatic people to allergen causes immediate bronchoconstriction, largely reflecting mast cell degranulation in the airways (called the early response), and a later phase of bronchoconstriction probably caused by secondary infiltration of inflammatory cells into the airways.

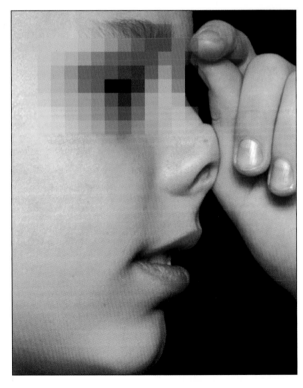

3.9 The 'allergic salute' of patients with atopic rhinitis caused by constant itchiness of the nose. Allergic rhinitis concomitant with asthma should always be enquired about, recognized and treated.

to obtain evidence of benefit of avoidance of perennial allergens, particularly house dust mite, in the asthmatic population as a whole[4]. This in part reflects the impracticability of performing blinded trials, the difficulty in achieving clinically relevant avoidance of many allergens and the fact that many patients with a positive skin prick test to any particular allergen do not have symptoms on allergen exposure and would therefore not benefit from avoidance. Ideally, avoidance measures should be restricted to allergen-reactive patients, which in the case of house dust mite can be established reliably only by provocation testing.

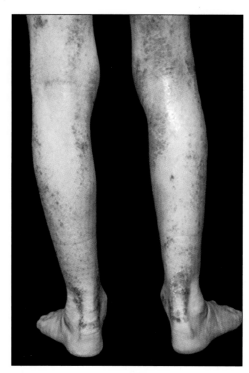

3.10 Atopic dermatitis, or eczema, is a common manifestation of the atopic diathesis that suggests the possibility of accompanying asthma, allergic rhinitis or food allergy.

Non-atopic asthma

The physician Rackeman first recognized the propensity of external agents (now recognized as allergens) to trigger symptoms in some people with asthma but not others in 1947. Nowadays, non-atopic or 'intrinsic' asthmatics are defined as those who have uniformly negative skin prick tests or blood tests for specific IgE[5].

The clinical distinction between atopic and non-atopic asthma has been ratified by modern epidemiological studies which have shown that increased age, female sex, the presence of chronic rhinosinusitis and more severe impairment of lung function are associated with an elevated chance of the patient being non-atopic. Identification of non-atopic asthma is important since it implies that allergen avoidance is not necessary for disease management, and also that asthma may possibly have arisen because of some occupational insult (see below). In terms of pathogenesis, the existence of non-atopic asthma is of interest since it implies that asthma may develop in the complete absence of IgE-mediated responses to external allergens, although the situation has been further complicated by recent observations that IgE may be manufactured locally in the bronchial mucosa of asthmatic people in the absence of circulating, allergen-specific IgE.

Aspirin-sensitive asthma

Aspirin-sensitive asthma is characterized by rapid exacerbation on exposure to aspirin (**3.11**) and related non-steroidal anti-inflammatory drugs[6]. The nasal mucosa, gut and skin may also be involved, causing rhinitis, gastrointestinal upset and urticaria/angioedema. Aspirin sensitivity is seen in approximately 10% of adults with asthma and commonly begins in middle age. The disease is slightly more common in females, but there is no relation with atopy. Aspirin-sensitive asthmatic people are over-represented in those presenting with life-threatening severe asthma attacks. They also tend to have aggressive, chronic rhinosinusitis causing recurrent nasal polyps (**3.12**).

Although the mechanism of aspirin sensitivity remains unclear, most investigators agree that it is not immuno-

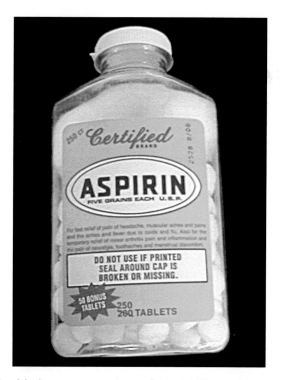

3.11 Aspirin is an extremely useful painkiller and antiplatelet agent, but in a minority (approximately 5–10%) of asthmatic people it may cause acute exacerbation of disease, chronic rhinosinusitis, gastrointestinal upset and urticaria.

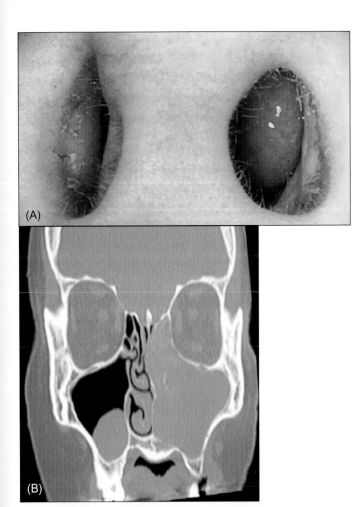

(A)

(B)

3.12 Nasal polyps appear as pinkish, anaesthetic protuberances into the nasal cavities. They may be caused by chronic allergic rhinitis or cystic fibrosis in children, but are particularly associated with aspirin-sensitive respiratory disease. (**A**) Clinical appearance. (**B**) Computed tomography scan showing complete occlusion of the left maxillary sinus.

logically mediated. There is no evidence of an IgE response to aspirin, and so the disease cannot be diagnosed by any immunological test, but only by experimental challenge and objective measurement of responses in the lungs or nasal cavities.

Aspirin-sensitive asthmatic people produce excess quantities of the cysteinyl leukotrienes LTC_4, LTD_4 and LTE_4 in the mucosa of the respiratory tract, reflected by the concentration of the stable end-product LTE_4 in the urine (**3.13**). Although aspirin-sensitive patients tend to have elevated urinary concentrations of LTE_4 even without aspirin exposure, this distinction is not sufficiently broad to be of diagnostic

use. Excessive cysteinyl leukotriene production in these patients may partly reflect genetic polymorphisms regulating the expression of enzymes controlling cysteinyl leukotriene synthesis, such as LTC_4 synthase, but may on the other hand simply reflect the fact that in general these patients have more severe airways inflammation. When aspirin-sensitive patients are challenged with aspirin, the production of cysteinyl leukotrienes is augmented, and this is thought to be responsible for the acute exacerbation of symptoms. One common characteristic of drugs exacerbating asthma in aspirin-sensitive patients is that they inhibit the enzyme cyclo-oxygenase-1 (COX-1), a widely expressed, constitutive enzyme responsible for the production of prostaglandins. Inhaled prostaglandin E_2 (PGE_2) inhibits bronchoconstriction in asthmatic people caused by exposure to allergens as well as aspirin, by 'braking' of leukotriene synthesis. Aspirin and other COX-1 inhibitors may therefore remove this 'braking' mechanism, but the question is why this does not cause acute bronchoconstriction in *all* asthmatic people. One possible reason is that aspirin-sensitive patients may have a critical deficiency in PGE_2 signalling[6].

There are several clinical implications arising from these observations. First, it is important to identify aspirin-sensitive patients. Aspirin sensitivity may be obvious from the history, or may require formal diagnosis by challenge with aspirin administered either orally or intranasally. Patients should be advised to avoid aspirin and other related COX-1 inhibitors, and make their problem widely known to medical and dental personnel. Some choose to wear personal warning pendants (**3.14**). Patients must use drugs other than aspirin for pain relief: most can tolerate paracetamol and drugs which inhibit the induced isoform of COX, or COX-2. These drugs do not, however, substitute for the antiplatelet activities of aspirin: alternative antiplatelet drugs must be employed if necessary.

Occupational asthma

Exposure to agents encountered and inhaled in the working environment is responsible for many chronic lung diseases including pulmonary fibrosis, extrinsic allergic alveolitis and occupational asthma. Continuous surveys of asthma arising in the workplace have currently implicated 147 different professions and 405 different compounds in the causation of occupational asthma (see McDonald *et al.*[7] and www.asmanet.com).

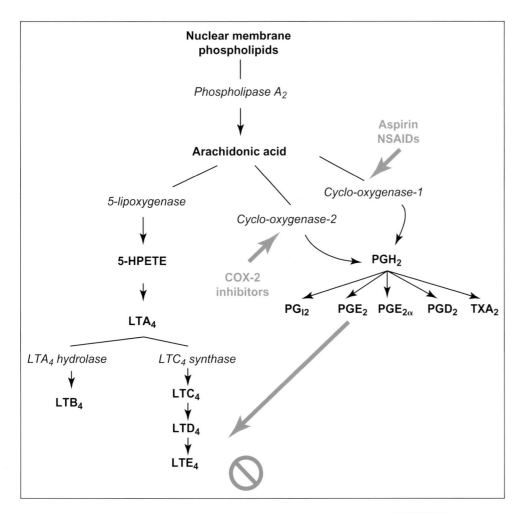

3.13 Overview of leukotriene and prostaglandin metabolism. Both mediators originate from arachidonic acid in the nuclear membrane of producing cells. Cyclo-oxygenase-1, inhibited by aspirin and related non-steroidal anti-inflammatory drugs (NSAIDs), reduces the production of prostaglandins. Prostaglandin E_2 (PGE_2) may play a critical role in 'braking' of the production of the cysteinyl leukotrienes LTC_4, LTD_4 and LTE_4. This 'braking' mechanism may be critically deficient in aspirin-sensitive asthmatic people, perhaps reflecting deficiencies in PGE_2 production and/or signalling in these patients.

Occupational asthma has increased progressively during the past few decades and is now the most prevalent occupational lung disease in many developed countries. Clinically, it may be defined as variable airways obstruction or bronchial hyper-responsiveness resulting from causes and conditions attributable to a particular working environment and not to stimuli encountered outside that environment. Epidemiological surveys suggest that the prevalence of occupational asthma is between 5% and 10% of the working population. The degree of individual exposure to the trigger factor is probably the most important risk factor. High molecular weight occupational sensitizers (typically proteins which act as allergens) are inhaled and most induce an IgE response. Some low molecular weight sensitizers, such as platinum salts, also induce specific IgE antibodies, probably by binding to endogenous body proteins as haptens thus forming new allergens. High molecular weight occupational agents and haptenated proteins may also directly stimulate T cells, which then precipitate

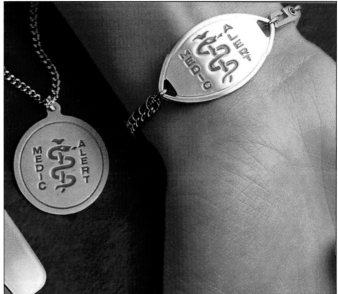

3.14 A personal warning pendant alerting medical and paramedical staff to a patient's aspirin sensitivity in the event of an unexpected emergency. Courtesy of The MedicAlert Foundation.

chronic bronchial inflammation. Such immunological responses to occupational agents are characterized by a period of latency. In other words, it typically takes 12–18 months for asthma to develop following the initiation of exposure. Symptoms of rhinoconjunctivitis often precede those of asthma. Clinical asthma arising from non-immunological mechanisms may also occur. The mechanism is uncertain, but may reflect direct damage of the bronchial epithelium by the sensitizing agent. This non-immunological form of occupational asthma is also known as reactive airways dysfunction syndrome. In theory any highly corrosive agent might cause reactive airways dysfunction syndrome but common culprits include acids, strong alkali such as ammonia and bleaches, gases such as sulphur dioxide, paint fumes and smoke.

Symptoms of asthma typically improve when affected patients are away from work and recur when they return (**3.15**). As exposure continues, symptoms occur earlier after exposure, and remission of symptoms may occur later, thus blurring the pattern of improvement away from work. Atopic subjects are much more prone to develop sensitization to high molecular weight agents where an IgE response is involved. Smoking further increases the risk. On the other hand, non-atopic subjects and non-smokers are more often affected by low molecular weight agents that do not induce an IgE response. An occupational

cause should be suspected in all new cases of adult-onset asthma, especially those patients who report worsening of their symptoms at work. Further investigation is best left in the hands of an experienced occupational physician. Guidelines are available for the preliminary diagnosis of occupational asthma by non-experts (see Vandenplas *et al.*[8] and www.occupationalasthma.com). Monitoring of the patient in the workplace, or experimental challenge may be necessary. Skin prick tests are available to detect IgE-mediated reactions to certain occupational sensitizing agents.

Exercise-induced asthma

Exercise is likely to exacerbate asthma in all patients (**3.16**) but this phenomenon is more prominent in some patients than others, which may partly reflect their lifestyle. It is a particularly worrying symptom for children during games, and athletes[9]. Exercise-induced asthma is more likely to occur in cold, dry environments. It is thought to reflect, as least partly, water loss from the airway wall which changes the local osmotic pressure, triggering degranulation of mast cells and perhaps activation of other inflammatory cells. The diagnosis can be made by formal exercise challenge, or less formally in children by measuring peak flow before

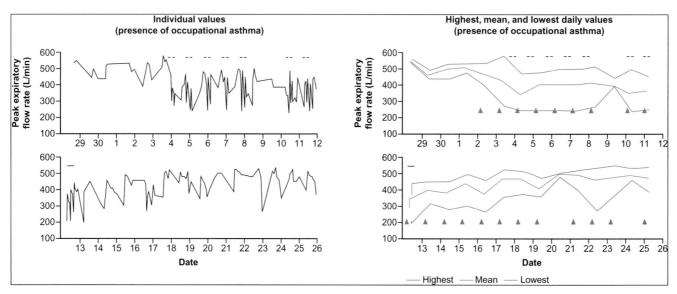

3.15 Pattern of changes in peak expiratory flow rate suggesting occupational asthma. The horizontal line shows a period of work; the triangles illustrate the need for an inhaled bronchodilator. Reproduced from Malo JL *et al.* (1993). How many times per day should the expiratory flow rate be assessed when investigating occupational asthma? *Thorax* **48**:1211–1217.

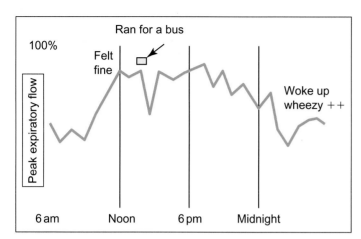

3.16 Exercise-induced asthma is a common everyday problem. Asthma symptoms may in some patients be entirely limited to exercise, but in others it is a reflection of poor overall asthma control. Simple everyday activities such as running for a bus can seriously upset asthma control in such patients.

and after they run up a few flights of stairs. Although bronchoconstriction may be strictly limited to exercise in some patients, it should be remembered that frequent exercise-induced symptoms are usually an indication of poor overall asthma control. This should prompt a complete review of overall symptoms, new exacerbating factors, and patient inhaler technique and compliance.

Asthma and infections

The common clinical impression, particularly in children, that viral infections (particularly infections with rhinovirus (**3.17**), respiratory syncytial virus and influenza virus) can trigger asthma has been confirmed by recent careful studies comparing variability in peak flow with proved viral infection[10] (**3.18**). The mechanism by which viruses exacerbate asthma is still not clear, but they may enhance the release of asthma-relevant mediators such as cytokines within the airways mucosa. Increased airways irritability resulting particularly in cough may be seen for weeks or even months after upper respiratory tract viral infections, even in non-asthmatic individuals, and whether or not the mechanism of this phenomenon is similar to that of exacerbation of established asthma, it is not hard to envisage how this post-viral irritability of the airways may be much more marked in asthmatic people.

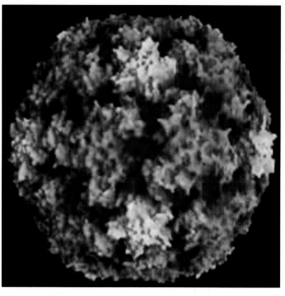

3.17 Upper respiratory tract viral infection is a common cause of disease exacerbation in asthmatic patients of all ages. From www.virology.net/Big_Virology/BVRNApicorna.html

Premenstrual asthma

In some women, particularly those with severe asthma, exacerbation of symptoms may occur premenstrually, typically 2 or 3 days before the onset of menstruation. This correlates with the late luteal phase of ovarian activity, when circulating oestrogens and progesterone reach their nadir at the end of the menstrual cycle. It is important to recognize this phenomenon. It is easily missed if not specifically enquired after. Again, marked premenstrual symptoms may reflect generalized poor control of asthma. Occasionally, blunting of the fall in progesterone by supplementation, or use of the oral contraceptive pill, may alleviate premenstrual asthma.

Therapy-resistant asthma

Asthma UK, the leading asthma lay charity estimates that, despite modern anti-asthma medications, up to 0.5 million asthmatic people in the UK (about 10% of the total) continue to suffer from chronic persistent symptoms. These patients lie at the extreme end of a spectrum of corticosteroid responsiveness, and often have severely impaired quality of life not only from their symptoms but also from the effects of excessive corticosteroid exposure.

3.18 Longitudinal studies documenting upper respiratory tract viral infections in asthmatics show that these commonly coincide with periods of asthma exacerbation. This is clearly shown in the peak flow records of three separate individuals followed through the summer and winter of the years 1989–1990.

The diagnosis of corticosteroid-resistant asthma is essentially one of exclusion. Before it can be made it must be ensured that the diagnosis of asthma is correct, that adequate dosages of corticosteroids are reaching the airways (compliance, inhaler technique, psychosocial factors detracting from compliance) and that factors contributing to poor asthma control (smoke, irritants, allergens, chronic rhinosinusitis, oesophageal reflux, drugs such as aspirin, β-blockers) have been eliminated as far as possible. This may involve prolonged assessment with management plans utilizing various inhaler devices and add-on therapies, with objective measurement of response. There is no universally accepted definition of corticosteroid resistance, but typically patients have:

- chronic airflow limitation (forced expiratory volume in one second [FEV_1] <60% predicted in adults and <80% predicted in children)
- frequent symptoms with diurnal variability of the peak expiratory flow
- poor clinical and spirometric response to systemic corticosteroid therapy, with <15% improvement in pre-bronchodilator FEV_1 following a trial of oral prednisolone therapy (at least 14 days of therapy with prednisolone or equivalent at a dosage of 40 mg/day) despite a typically brisk FEV_1 response to bronchodilator[11].

Such patients are tolerant of corticosteroid withdrawal, in contrast to corticosteroid-'dependent' patients who may not show a marked acute response to systemic corticosteroid but rapidly deteriorate when such therapy is withdrawn. Nevertheless both resistant and dependent patients probably lie towards the far end of the same spectrum of corticosteroid responsiveness.

Corticosteroids have many anti-inflammatory effects but a key facet of their anti-asthma activity is thought to be inhibition of T cell activation and cytokine production. Congruently, there is evidence that T cells from corticosteroid-resistant asthmatic people are refractory to the inhibitory effects of corticosteroid both *in vitro* and *in vivo* (reviewed by Corrigan and Lee[12]). Evidence suggests that this refractoriness may be acquired in a number of different ways involving dysregulation of intracellular signalling mediators which interact with, or act on the ligand-bound corticosteroid receptor, altering its ability to trans-repress cytokine gene expression[12]. For example, the transcriptional element activator protein (AP)-1, which increases transcrip-

tion of many asthma-relevant cytokines such as interleukin (IL)-4, IL-5 and IL-13, and which can bind to and inactivate the ligand-bound corticosteroid receptor, appears to be overexpressed in T cells from corticosteroid-resistant asthmatic people. The stimulus for this overexpression is unknown, but oxidative stress (from smoking or poor dietary antioxidant intake) is one possibility. Other signalling pathways such as mitogen-activated or extracellular signal-regulated protein kinase (MEK)/extracellular signal-regulated protein kinase (ERK), activated by enterotoxin superantigens from *Staphylococcus aureus*, and p38 mitogen-activated protein (MAP) kinase have been shown to phosphorylate the corticosteroid receptor itself, altering its abilities to bind corticosteroid and translocate to the cell nucleus. It will be some time before this immense complexity of interactions is fully elucidated, but already these early findings suggest new strategies for clinical characterization of asthmatic people (smoking, dietary antioxidant intake, bacterial colonization of the airways) better to predict their responsiveness to corticosteroid therapy.

In the meantime, these patients are difficult to manage. In clinical practice, because there is little hard evidence to justify withdrawing corticosteroid therapy from resistant patients, this process is often ignored or delayed while unwanted effects of the therapy accumulate. Trials of alternative 'immunosuppressive' drugs such as ciclosporin, methotrexate and gold salts in these patients[12] have been generally unsatisfactory in the sense that many patients fail to respond and it is impossible to predict responsiveness *a priori*. Furthermore, chronic immunosuppression begets the spectre of serious infection or malignancy, and there is in addition a not insignificant list of possible problems associated, in some patients, with the use of each particular drug. It is to be hoped that better understanding of the likely many mechanisms involved in therapy resistance in asthma will allow better targeted and more successful alternative therapeutic approaches, including perhaps modification of environmental influences.

References

1. Corrigan CJ, Rak S (2004). *Rapid Reference Allergy*. Elsevier Mosby, London, Chapters 1, 2.
2. Taylor PE, Jonsson H (2004). Thunderstorm asthma. *Curr Allergy Asthma Rep*, 4:409–413.

3. Sherrill D, Stein R, Kurzius-Spencer M, Martinez F (1999). Early sensitisation to allergens and development of respiratory symptoms. *Clin Exp Allergy*, **29**:905–11.

4. Gotzsche PC, Johansen HK, Burr ML, Hammarquist C (2001). House dust mite control measures for asthma (Cochrane Review). In: *The Cochrane Library*. Issue 3. Update Software, Oxford.

5. Corrigan C (2004). Mechanisms of intrinsic asthma. *Curr Opin Allergy Clin Immunol*, **4**:53–56.

6. Ying S, Corrigan CJ, Lee TH (2004). Mechanisms of aspirin sensitive asthma. *Allergol Int*, **53**:111–119.

7. McDonald JC, Chen Y, Zekveld C, Cherry NM (2005). Incidence by occupation and industry of acute work related respiratory diseases in the UK, 1992–2001. *Occup Environ Med*, **62**:836–842.

8. Vandenplas O, Ghezzo H, Munoz X, Moscato G, Perfetti L, Lemiere C, Labrecque M, L'Archeveque J, Malo JL (2005). What are the questionnaire items most useful in identifying subjects with occupational asthma? *Eur Respir J*, **26**:1056–1063.

9. Milgrom H (2004). Exercise-induced asthma: ways to wise exercise. *Curr Opin Allergy Clin Immunol*, **4**:147–153.

10. Johnston SL (2005). Overview of virus-induced airway disease. *Proc Am Thorac Soc*, **2**:150–156.

11. Lee TH, Brattsand R, Leung D (1996). Corticosteroid action and resistance in asthma. *Am J Respir Crit Care Med*, **154**:S51.

12. Corrigan CJ, Lee TH (2005). Glucocorticoid action and resistance in asthma. *Allergol Int*, **54**:235–243.

Chapter 4

Aetiology of Asthma

Gwyneth A Davies and Julian M Hopkin

Introduction

The origins of asthma are multifactorial, and it arises from a complex interaction of genetic and environmental factors. Genetic factors underlie the population *susceptibility* to asthma which is then induced by particular environmental stimuli. Genetic variation may influence asthma at a number of levels such as resistance of the bronchial epithelial barrier to insult (e.g. allergen, virus); T helper (Th)2 immunity (upregulated in asthma and atopy); and response of the whole airway to injury (relevant to airway remodelling).

Atopy is the main predictor of asthma between the ages of 5 and 25 years, and is a Th2 cell driven hypersensitivity to innocuous antigens (allergens), clinically manifested by epithelial inflammation. However, atopy is not synonymous with asthma, which occurs without atopy in up to 30% of cases.

The reasons for the recent impressive rise in asthma and atopy in Westernised countries are as yet unclear. It is likely that relevant environmental factors are exerting an influence early in life, in those with genetic predisposition. Theories include changes in microbial exposure in childhood, house dust mite sensitization, diet and air pollution.

Genetic susceptibility

Human chromosomes

Asthma clusters in families and first-degree relatives of asthmatic people have a significantly higher prevalence of asthma than relatives of non-asthmatic people. Twin studies estimate the proportion of asthma due to genetic variation to be 50–60%. Genome-wide screens have shown repeatable linkages of chromosomal regions with asthma and related traits of bronchial hyper-responsiveness (BHR) and atopy (total IgE levels, IgE to specific allergens, skin prick tests) (**4.1, 4.2**). The most replicated linkages are to the following regions: 2p; 4q; 5q23-31; 6p24-21; 11q13-21; 12q21-24; 13q12-14; 16p12; 16q21-23; and 19q[1,2]. Most of these chromosomal regions contain hundreds of genes, many of them potential asthma-susceptibility genes. For instance, the 5q region – implicated in phenotypes ranging from asthma and BHR to total IgE levels – contains the cytokine gene cluster and the gene coding for the β_2-adrenergic receptor (**4.3**).

Major genes in asthma, BHR, IgE/atopy

Asthma is a polygenic disease. Variants in 80 genes have been associated with asthma or related traits, but it is likely that only a few genes are important, with several common variants each exerting a modest functional effect (**4.4**).

Genes associated with asthma and related traits include the cytokine cluster on chromosome 5 (interleukin (IL)-4, IL-13, IL-9, IL-5, CD14 and β_2-adrenergic receptor); the human leucocyte antigen (HLA) and tumour necrosis factor (TNF) genes on chromosome 6; the β chain of the high affinity IgE receptor and the Clara cell secretory protein on chromosome 11; and the α chain of the IL-4 receptor on chromosome 16[2]. Associations are often not replicated in other populations, implying that different populations have different asthma characteristics associated with particular genetic markers.

Good examples of widely replicated associations are the genes coding for the IL-4/IL-13 pathway. This makes biological sense as IL-4 and IL-13 are important Th2 cytokines, central to the bronchial inflammation seen in asthma, with actions including isotype switching to IgE. Asthma/atopy phenotypes have been associated not only with variants in

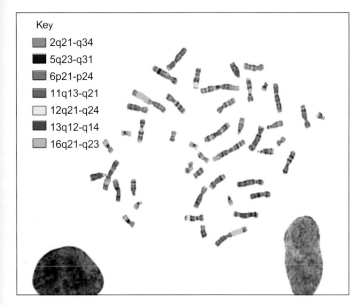

Key
- ▦ 2q21-q34
- ■ 5q23-q31
- ▦ 6p21-p24
- ▦ 11q13-q21
- ▫ 12q21-q24
- ▦ 13q12-q14
- ▦ 16q21-q23

4.1 Asthma is both *polygenic* and *genetically heterogeneous.* That is, many genes can contribute to asthma and the combination of genes is different in different families. Highlighted on this diploid set of human chromosomes are the most widely replicated regions of 'linkage' with asthma and related traits. There are two main methods of examining the genetic basis of complex diseases such as asthma: genome screens and candidate-gene studies. Genome screens apply a random approach, using panels of DNA markers distributed uniformly across the genome, to identify which chromosomal regions are co-inherited ('linked') with disease. In the candidate-gene approach, a gene is chosen on the basis of its functional relevance, and variants of the gene are then tested for their association with asthma. In practice, both approaches may be integrated as genome screens identify relatively large areas of linkage. Fine mapping of the region and positional cloning is needed to actually identify the gene of interest. These approaches have been successfully employed to identify novel asthma-susceptibility genes (*ADAM33, DPP10, PHF11, GPRA*). Image courtesy of Dr Shareen H Doak, School of Medicine, University of Wales Swansea.

the IL-4/IL-13 genes themselves, but also in their common receptor (IL-4Ra) and transcription factor STAT6 (**4.5, 4.6**). Interactions between these variants increase the risk of asthma and atopy further. The IL-13 Gln110 variant reduces binding to a decoy receptor, with resultant increased IL-13

levels seen in asthmatic people, demonstrating its functional effect (**4.7**)[3].

Five novel candidate genes have been identified by positional cloning strategies over the past 3 years. These fine-mapping techniques allow progress from broad chromosomal linkage regions to gene identification (**4.8**). These genes (*ADAM33, DPP110, PHF11, GPRA, HLA-G*) are not involved in known asthma pathways. These genetic studies offer new insights into asthma pathogenesis, suggesting that pathways relating to tissue growth and remodelling may be important.

The genetic contribution to asthma is complex and involves polygenic inheritance and genetic heterogeneity (different combinations of genes causing asthmatic traits in different individuals). Gene–gene and gene–environment interactions underpin the aetiology of asthma, the complexity of which is just beginning to be unravelled.

Environmental factors

Migrants moving to Western countries have an increased risk of acquiring asthma, emphasizing the importance of environment in disease development. Maternal asthma confers a greater risk of asthma than paternal asthma, and Th2 skewing occurs in cord blood in atopy, suggesting that the *in-utero* environment may account for later asthma[4, 5]. Since the recent rise in asthma and atopy in the developed world has occurred over a matter of decades, environmental factors must be responsible – but which environmental factors have driven the rising prevalence in asthma?

Common allergens
Allergens are defined as antigens that promote IgE sensitization. They are diverse in origin and character and unified by their resistance to heat and protein digestion. They can act as proteases (house dust mite antigens); non-specific lipid transfer proteins (certain food allergens); or gelsolins that interfere with the actin cytoskeleton of cells. Allergens important in asthma are common antigens which are efficiently delivered into the airways within respired particles. Allergen proteases can trigger epithelial cells directly or via protein activating receptors (especially proteinase-activated receptor (PAR)-2), releasing Th2 cytokines and chemokines.

House dust mite accounts for the highest sensitization rates in the UK, followed by cat and grass pollen. Other

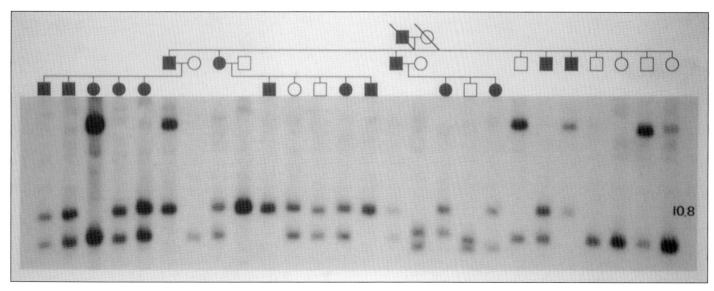

4.2 Family tree of the first family showing linkage of atopy with chromosome 11q. Family members with atopy are shown in black. The 10.8 kb band is *inherited* in family members *with atopy* but *not inherited* in those *without atopy* in 20 of 23 cases. The band is on chromosome 11q, suggesting the importance of this region in the inheritance of atopy, confirmed in later studies.

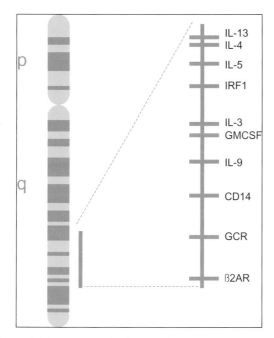

4.3 The cytokine gene cluster on chromosome 5q31-q33. This region contains several genes with well-replicated associations with asthma. The region is exceptional in that here a number of loci contribute to asthma susceptibility. Generally, one major locus for asthma susceptibility is identified from a chromosomal region of interest e.g. *ADAM33* on chromosome 20p. IL, interleukin; IRF, interleukin regulatory factor; GMCSF, granulocyte macrophage colony stimulating factor; GCR, glucocorticoid receptor; β2AR, β2 adrenergic receptor.

common aeroallergens include tree pollens, dog, and the moulds *Aspergillus fumigatus* and *Alternaria alternata* (**4.9**). In the humid south-eastern American states, cockroach sensitization is more common.

Role of allergen sensitization

Allergens penetrate the mucosal epithelial lining where they induce the allergic response. Sensitization is defined by positive skin prick tests (**4.10**) or specific IgE directed against common allergens. Early allergic sensitization, particularly to indoor allergens, is a major risk factor for the development of asthma in genetically susceptible individuals (**4.11, 4.12**). House dust mite sensitization is a significant risk factor for the development of asthma, hayfever and eczema[4, 5]. Furthermore, sensitization to common aeroallergens is associated with increased BHR.

The highest risk of childhood asthma has been seen in children sensitized very early in life. However, this was only true for children with a family history of asthma/atopy leading to speculation about whether the relation between allergic sensitization and asthma is actually causal or represents parallel pathways arising from common genetic origins.

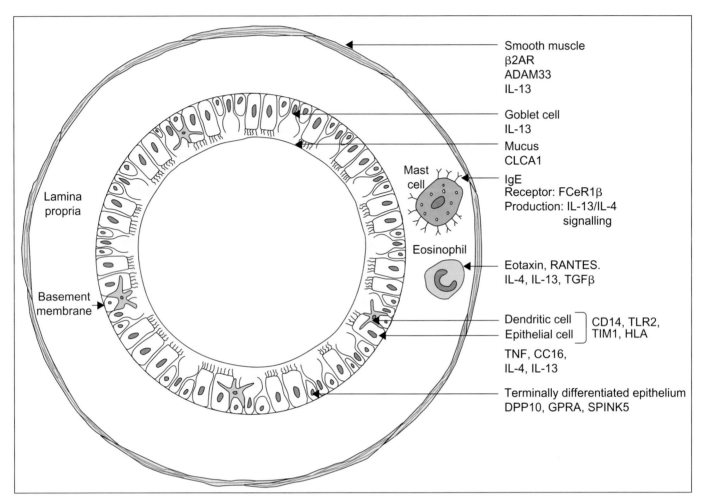

4.4 Polygenic nature of asthma: variants at a number of genes affect bronchial function. This airway diagram shows proteins encoded by asthma-susceptibility genes. These proteins may have a multitude of actions. The T helper (Th)2 cytokine interleukin (IL)-13 causes bronchoconstriction; mucus hypersecretion; and acts with IL-4 to influence IgE production. Human leucocyte antigen (HLA) and microbial pattern recognition receptors (CD14, TLR2, TIM1) are widely expressed. The function of the positionally cloned genes *DPP10*, *GPRA* and *SPINK5*, present in the terminally differentiated epithelium, is as yet unknown. *ADAM33* is thought to influence bronchial hyper-responsiveness. ADAM, a disintegrin and metalloproteinase; CLCA, calcium-dependent chloride channel; STAT, signal transducer and activator of transcription; RANTES, regulated upon activation, normally T-expressed and secreted; TGF, transforming growth factor; TLR, toll-like receptor; TIM, T cell immunoglobulin and mucin containing molecules; CC, Clara cell; TNF, tumour necrosis factor; DPP, dipeptidyl peptidase; GPRA, G-protein-coupled receptor for asthma susceptibility; SPINK5, serine protease inhibitor, kazal type 5.

Aetiology of asthma 41

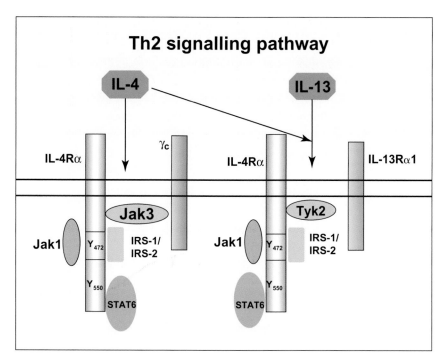

Th2 signalling pathway

4.5 Interleukin (IL)-4 and IL-13 are important Th2 cytokines and are central to the bronchial inflammation seen in asthma. IL-4 and IL-13 share a common receptor, the α chain of the IL-4 receptor (IL4Rα). Phosphorylation of the kinases (Jak, Janus kinase; Tyk, tyrosine kinase) and IRS (insulin receptor substrate) causes activation of STAT6, signal transducer and activator of transcription which transmits the signal to the nucleus.

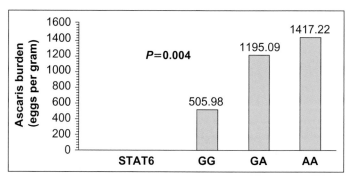

4.6 The evolutionary origin of asthma. Genetic variants associated with asthma may have their origin in protecting against parasitic infestation. The graph shows that a child's parasitic burden (ascaris egg count) is influenced by their genotype. The genotype GG of STAT6, a predictor of asthma, shows lower egg counts compared with GA and AA[13]. The marked Th2 immune response seen in asthma is also the body's natural response against parasites, with increased IgE production and eosinophilia.

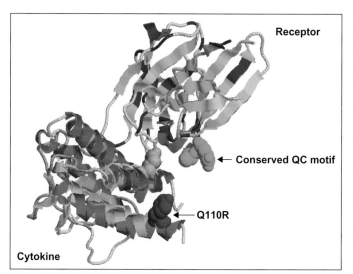

4.7 Molecular model of the interleukin (IL)-13 cytokine-receptor complex. Individual genetic variants have modest functional effects in asthma. It is the combination of modest effects at a number of loci that confer susceptibility to disease. For example, experiments show diminished binding of an IL-13 variant to a decoy receptor, with resultant higher levels of IL-13 seen in asthmatics[5]. This is due to the interaction between the altered amino acid (Q110R, above) and a conserved motif on the receptor – shown here in a molecular model. Molecular modelling courtesy of Dr Jonathan Mullins, School of Medicine, University of Wales Swansea.

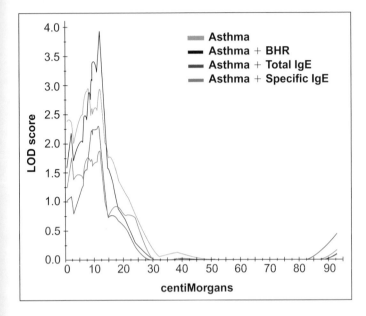

4.8 The importance of defining different phenotypes in asthma. The figure shows a linkage analysis of chromosome 20 with different asthma phenotypes, which led to the identification of *ADAM33* as the locus of interest. Variation at the *ADAM33* locus was found to influence bronchial hyper-responsiveness (BHR). Note the relatively weaker signal when examining the locus with relation to asthma and total IgE levels compared to the much stronger signal when looking at the combination of BHR and asthma. Adapted from Van Eerdewegh P *et al.* (2002). Association of the ADAM33 gene with asthma and bronchial hyperresponsiveness. *Nature*, **418**(6896):426–430.

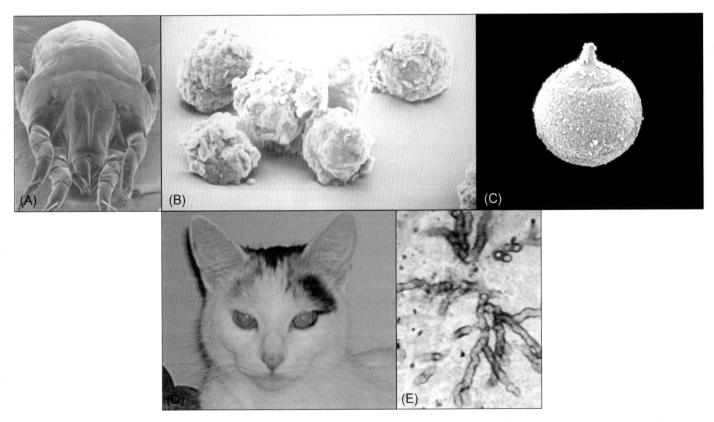

4.9 Common allergens. (**A**) House dust mite, which thrives in modern centrally heated homes (photo courtesy of Enrique Fernández-Caldas, Madrid). The allergens *Der p 1* and *Der p 2* are potent proteases contained in the mite's faecal pellets (**B**). (**C**) Pollens from grasses, birch and ragwort are an important source of allergens (Japanese cedar pollen grain shown here). (**D**) Cats' saliva contains the allergen *Fel d 1* which is transferred to its fur during grooming, and which becomes widespread throughout the home so that cat sensitization can occur even without direct animal contact. (**E**) The mould *Aspergillus fumigatus* releases its allergenic spores in the winter season.

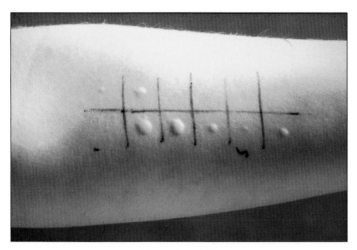

4.10 Positive skin prick tests: a common feature of asthma in children and young adults. An intradermal injection of purified allergen is used. When allergen specific IgE is present, it binds to skin mast cells and cross-linking of adjacent IgE molecules by allergen causes mast cell degranulation with release of inflammatory mediators. A wheal and flare reaction is seen within minutes. The test is judged positive if the wheal is 3 mm greater than the saline control after 15 minutes.

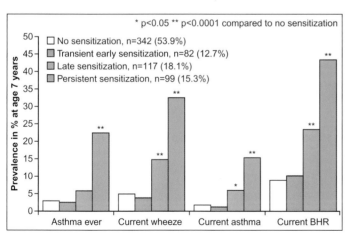

4.11 Persistent sensitization to allergen is a strong predictor of asthma and BHR. The bar chart shows the prevalence of asthma and asthmatic symptoms at age 7 years, stratified for sensitization pattern. Asthma and associated traits are associated with a strikingly higher prevalence of persistent sensitization compared with no sensitization. From Illi S *et al.* (2001). The pattern of atopic sensitization is associated with the development of asthma in childhood. *J Allergy Clin Immunol*, **108**:709–714.

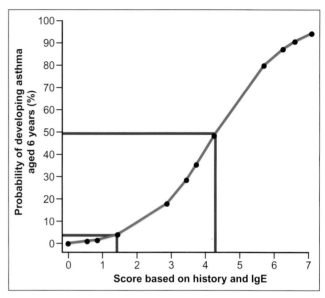

4.12 Sensitization to aeroallergens is a useful predictor of asthma in later childhood. This graph illustrates how the addition of specific IgE to a clinical scoring system (derived from 3–4 year olds, wheezing, familial allergy for pollen) considerably refines the prediction of which child will develop asthma. Straight lines represent 3-year-old child with a family history after a negative (1) and positive (2) IgE test (cat, dog and/or house dust mite). IgE: immunoglobulin E. From Eyesink PED *et al.* (2005). Accuracy of specific IgE in the prediction of asthma: development of a scoring formula for general practice. *Br J Gen Pract*, **55**:125–131.

Role of allergen exposure

The development of allergen sensitization requires exposure to that allergen. Once sensitization has occurred, repeated exposure to that allergen is likely to trigger symptoms. Although house dust mite levels are related to mite sensitization and wheezy illness, rising house dust mite levels are not felt to account for the general increased prevalence of atopic disease. Asthma prevalence has also risen in hot dry areas where mite levels are low. It seems unlikely that increased allergen exposure accounts for the rise in atopy, since sensitization to all allergens has increased simultaneously, suggesting a generally heightened allergic response. Higher allergen exposure may mean more sensitization to that allergen, but this does not necessarily translate into increased childhood asthma (**4.13**)[4].

Having a cat or dog at home may actually be protective against the development of atopy and wheeze. Hence the

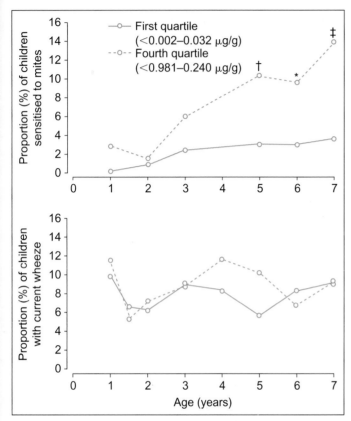

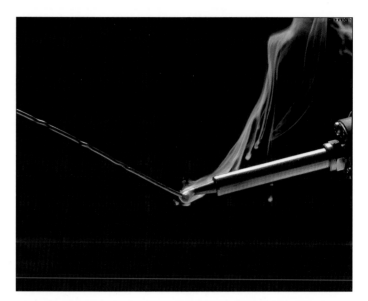

4.14 Soldering fumes can cause occupational asthma. Flux cored solder is used in the electronics industry and contains colophony, a natural product derived from pine resin. Colophony fumes released from solder flux during soldering can cause asthma and colophony is also a well-recognized skin sensitizer. Courtesy of Purex International Ltd.

4.13 Level of allergen exposure is a strong determinant of early sensitization in childhood but there is no clear evidence of a direct link between exposure and asthma. The graphs show that house dust mite allergen exposure is related to specific sensitization but not to prevalence of wheezing at age 1–7 years. From Lau S *et al.* (2000). Early exposure to house-dust mite and cat allergens and development of childhood asthma: a cohort study. *Lancet*, **356**:1392–1397.

relation between allergen exposure and asthma is far from being completely resolved. Although cats have been shown to be *protective* against wheeze in children *without* a maternal history of asthma, risk of wheeze was *increased* in those *with* a maternal history, indicating the importance of gene–environment interactions[6].

Finally, primary prevention studies involving reduction of house dust mite exposure have been disappointing. Allergen exposure is not a proven risk factor for childhood asthma. Allergen exposure may increase the risk of atopic disease, but outcome is highly dependent on dose, type of allergen, age at exposure and host susceptibility.

Table 4.1 Commonest agents and occupations implicated in occupational asthma*

Agents	Occupations
• Isocyanates	• Industrial workers e.g. paint-sprayers
• Flour	• Bakers/pastry makers
• Colophony/fluxes	• Electronics workers/welders
• Latex	• Hospital/laboratory workers
• Aldehydes	• Chemical/wood workers
• Enzymes	• Detergent manufacturers
• Animals	• Animal handlers
• Wood dusts	• Timber workers

*Agents can be divided into reactive chemicals (e.g. isocyanates) and organic antigens (e.g. wheat flour). Organic antigens induce IgE sensitization. Reactive chemicals act in various ways, e.g. acid anhydrides are haptens and need to bind to native proteins to induce an IgE response.

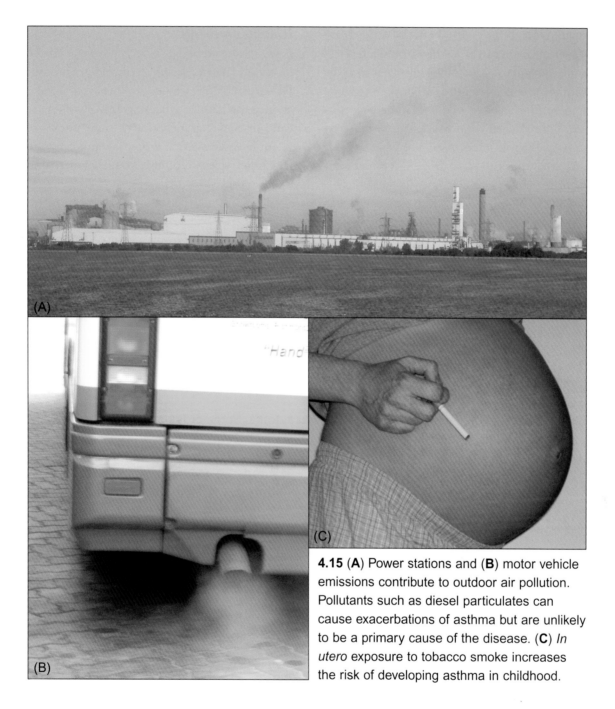

4.15 (A) Power stations and **(B)** motor vehicle emissions contribute to outdoor air pollution. Pollutants such as diesel particulates can cause exacerbations of asthma but are unlikely to be a primary cause of the disease. **(C)** *In utero* exposure to tobacco smoke increases the risk of developing asthma in childhood.

Occupational asthma

Occupational irritants can worsen pre-existing asthma. Occupational asthma *per se* is asthma caused by exposure to a particular occupational agent (*Table 4.1*, **4.14**). These agents can be divided into reactive chemicals (e.g. isocyantes) or organic antigens (e.g. wheat flour). For both, the pathological and physiological changes in the airway are similar, but the mechanisms underlying the development can be different. Organic antigens promote IgE response. Reactive chemicals act in various ways – the acid anhydrides produce haptens with native proteins, resulting in IgE production to these complexes. The mechanism for the highly reactive isocyanates remains unclear. High exposures to occupational agents increase the risk of asthma. Other risk factors interact, e.g. smoking increases the risk of isocyanate occupational asthma. Pre-existent atopy predisposes to occupational asthma from organic antigens (e.g. flour). HLA class 2 variation influences risk of response to reactive chemicals (e.g. DQB1 for isocyantes, DRB1 for Western Red Cedar).

Role of air pollution

Air pollutants such as ozone can exacerbate asthma. It is less clear whether air pollutants – including nitrogen dioxide, ozone, sulphur dioxide and particulate carbons – contribute to the development of asthma (**4.15**)[7]. Declining air pollution in Western industrialized countries has occurred concurrently with increasing asthma prevalence which argues against a strong effect on asthma causation. Asthma rates were lower in former East Germany (with greater air pollution) compared with West Germany, with similar findings from large surveys elsewhere.

Pollution is unlikely to be a primary cause of asthma but epidemiological and experimental evidence suggests that diesel exhaust particulates and ozone promote allergen sensitization. Individuals with particular genotypes related to antioxidant defences (e.g. glutathione S-transferase variants) may be more susceptible to the effects of pollution[7].

Role of smoking

Exposure to tobacco smoke *in utero* is associated with increased risk of allergic sensitization and asthma (**4.15C**). Passive smoking – especially maternal smoking – confers an increased risk of wheezing and/or asthma at least until a child reaches 7 years and active smoking increases the risk of adult-onset wheeze. If the father also smokes, the risk of childhood wheeze increases but maternal smoking confers the greatest risk[4, 5].

Role of diet

Change in the Western diet, with reduced intake of antioxidants, has led to speculation on the role of nutrients (including antioxidant vitamins, omega-3 fatty acids, selenium, magnesium, sodium and zinc). Some cross-sectional studies support an association but there is no conclusive evidence (*Table 4.2*)[8].

Table 4.2 Summary of evidence on the role of nutrients in asthma. Some cross-sectional studies support an association between reduced antioxidant intake and asthma but there is little evidence that diet plays a major role in asthma causation

Nutrient	Cross-sectional	Case–control	Longitudinal	Interventional
Vitamin C	Reduced risk of asthma Mixed results	Protective Mixed results	No effect on asthma incidence	Limited evidence of protection, given with other antioxidants
Vitamin E	No effect	Protective Mixed results	Limited evidence of protection	Limited evidence of protection, given with other antioxidants
Vitamin A or β-carotene	Inconclusive	Protective Mixed results	No effect on asthma incidence	Limited evidence of protection, given with other antioxidants
ω-3 fatty acids	N/A	Limited evidence of protection	No effect on asthma incidence	Protective Mixed results
Selenium	No effect	Protective	N/A	No effect
Magnesium	Protective	Protective	N/A	No effect
Sodium	Mostly no effect	Limited evidence of increased airway reactivity	N/A	Some evidence of increased risk

N/A, not available.

Early life studies show breastfeeding to reduce eczema but remain inconclusive regarding protection against asthma. Diet in pregnancy may affect the developing immune system and ω-3 fatty acid supplementation has shown beneficial effects[5, 8].

An 'obesity epidemic' has paralleled the rise in asthma in the Western world. Is there a causal link? An increased prevalence of asthma is seen in overweight individuals, especially women. Weight loss trials have shown a reduction in asthma signs and symptoms but may be confounded by related factors of diet and physical activity[9].

Role of infection

'Hygiene hypothesis'

The pattern of microbial exposure in childhood has changed considerably in Western countries, as a result of a cleaner environment, widespread antibiotic use and immunizations. The 'hygiene hypothesis' suggests that lack of exposure to childhood infection, endotoxin and microbial products causes persistence of Th2 responses, thus increasing the likelihood of atopic disease[10, 11].

Observations supporting the hygiene hypothesis are that asthma and atopy are:

- less common in children with more siblings or in those attending daycare, presumably due to increased exposure to childhood infections (**4.16**)
- strikingly less common in children living on livestock farms, who have a higher exposure to endotoxins (**4.17**)
- commoner in Western countries.

Further refinements to the hygiene hypothesis stem from the suggestion that specific infections occurring at critical times in immune development are most important:

- *Mycobacterial infection.* Some epidemiological studies have suggested an inverse relation between mycobacterial exposure and asthma/atopy.
- *Intestinal flora.* The gut is a critical regulator of the immune response and adequate intestinal flora may be important in guarding against atopy. This is supported by the association between enteric infection (hepatitis A), family size and absence of atopy in Italian recruits[12]. Probiotics studies have yielded some encouraging results.
- *Helminth infection* (**4.18**). The Th2 response forms the basis of the natural immune response against parasites, with increased IgE production and eosinophilia. Interestingly,

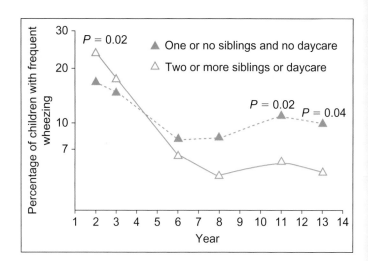

4.16 The hygiene hypothesis: children with greater exposure to other children – and thus more infections – have a *reduced* risk of asthma symptoms in later childhood. The graph shows that children exposed to more siblings/daycare had more wheeze at age 2 years but their risk of wheezing dropped after the age of 4 years and was significantly decreased beginning at age 11 years. Redrawn from Ball TM *et al.* (2000). Exposure to siblings and day care during infancy and subsequent development of asthma and frequent wheeze. *N Eng J Med*, **343**:538–543.

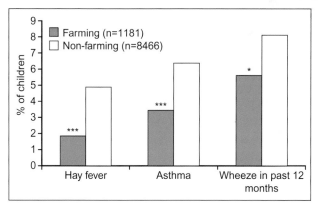

4.17 Protective effect of living on a farm: shown here by prevalence of atopic disease in children of farming (filled bars) and non-farming parents (unfilled bars). Children living on a farm had a significantly lower prevalence (%) of hay fever, asthma and wheeze than children not living on a farm. The protective effect of the farming environment may be due to increased exposure to endotoxin and microbial products. Adapted from data in von Ehrenstein OS *et al.* (2000). Reduced risk of hay fever and asthma among children of farmers. *Clin Exp Allergy*, **30**:87–93.

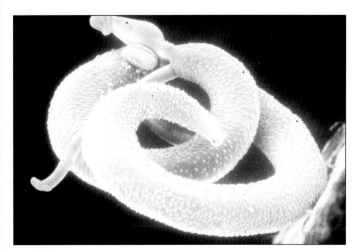

4.18 The helminth *Schistosoma mansoni*. The T helper (Th)2 response (with eosinophilia and IgE production) is the body's natural defence mechanism against parasitic infestations such as worms. When directed against innocuous environmental antigens, the Th2 response can lead to asthma and atopic disease. Paradoxically, helminth infestation seems to be protective against asthma. Helminths switch on production of the regulatory cytokine IL-10 which may switch off Th2 responses to innocuous environmental antigens.

worm infestation appears to be protective against asthma despite the marked Th2 response common to both[13]. Moreover, antihelminthic treatment appears to increase allergen sensitization. One explanation is that helminths stimulate exuberant IL-10 production which reduces specific IgE to aeroallergens, thus causing deviation away from an atopic phenotype.

Role of viruses

The sensitive method of reverse transcriptase-DNA amplification, detecting viruses in respiratory materials, emphasizes the role of viral infections in exacerbations of asthma (85% in children, 70% in adults). Asthmatic respiratory epithelial cells appear more susceptible to viruses, although it is unclear whether this is a primary epithelial defect or the result of Th2-induced inflammatory damage. Viral infection promotes further inflammation in the airway – with prominent actions from nuclear factor κB and activator protein (AP)-1, and specific enhancement of Th2-induced inflammation by CD8+ T lymphocytes and chemokines CCL3 and CCL5.

It has been suggested that viral infections, in particular respiratory syncytial virus (RSV), act as an independent risk factor for asthma and atopy (**4.19**). Bronchiolitis associated with other viruses may be associated with an even greater risk of childhood asthma[14]. This would appear to contradict the hygiene hypothesis which suggests childhood infections to be protective against the development of asthma. However, since RSV infection is almost universal by the age of 2 years, host susceptibility must play a part in which children go on to develop asthma. Fascinating interactions between genes and environment may explain these apparent paradoxes, e.g. differential responses of specific genotypes to viral infections and daycare[15]. Another explanation is that viral infection with wheeze acts as a marker for asthma and reflects impaired viral handling by the asthmatic lung[14]. Studies are ongoing to answer this intriguing question.

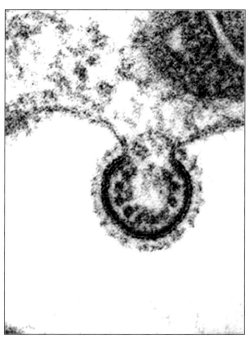

4.19 Electron micrograph of respiratory syncytial virus (RSV), budding. Early viral infection with wheeze predicts subsequent childhood wheeze and has been implicated as a risk factor for asthma. Since RSV infection is almost universal by the age of 2 years, it is unclear whether infection is a causal factor for asthma or a marker of disease, representing impaired viral handling by the allergic lung. Image courtesy of Professor R P Garofalo, University of Texas Medical Branch, Galveston, Texas, USA; Author, Asma Al-Thani.

Role of the epithelial mesenchymal trophic unit

Although the central role of Th2 inflammation is undisputed, bronchial remodelling represents a crucial component of bronchial hyper-reactivity in established asthma, and is an important cause of declining lung function with time. This remodelling includes epithelial goblet cell hyperplasia, thickening of the basement membrane by collagen deposition and smooth muscle hypertrophy (**4.20**). Is it simply the result of chronic Th2 inflammation or has it a more primary causation? The interaction between epithelium and mesenchyme is exemplified by transforming growth factor β_2 release from injured or stimulated epithelial cells, which acts on fibroblasts to cause myofibroblast development and smooth muscle hypertrophy. Variants of ADAM33 (a zinc-dependent metalloprotease) are strongly linked with bronchial reactivity, and this protein is specifically expressed in smooth muscle and myofibroblasts – therefore innate susceptibility within the mesenchyme may be a primary disposer towards remodelling. Hence the epithelium and the mesenchyme together play important mechanistic roles in asthma, complementing Th2 immune mechanisms and IgE sensitization.

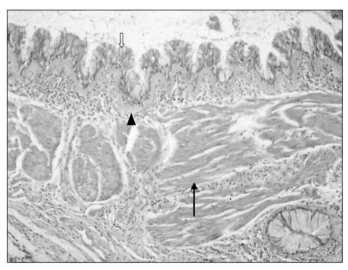

4.20 Airway remodelling, demonstrated on histological section of an asthmatic airway. There is marked thickening of the basement membrane (arrowhead), smooth muscle hypertrophy (closed arrow) and goblet cell hyperplasia (open arrow). With thanks to Professor Stephen Holgate, University of Southampton.

References

1. Wills-Karp M, Ewart SL (2004). Time to draw breath: asthma-susceptibility genes are identified. *Nat Rev Genet*, **5**(5):376–387.
2. Ober C, Hoffjan S (2006). Asthma genetics 2006: the long and winding road to gene discovery. *Genes Immun*, **7**(2):95–100.
3. Arima K, Umeshita-Suyama R, Sakata Y, Akaiwa M, Mao XQ, Enomoto T, Dake Y, Shimazu S, Yamashita T, Sugawara N, Brodeur S, Geha R, Puri RK, Sayegh MH, Adra CN, Hamasaki N, Hopkin JM, Shirakawa T, Izuhara K (2002). Upregulation of IL-13 concentration in vivo by the IL13 variant associated with bronchial asthma. *J Allergy Clin Immunol*, **109**(6):980–987.
4. von Mutius E (2002). Environmental factors influencing the development and progression of pediatric asthma. *J Allergy Clin Immunol*, **109**(6 Suppl):S525–532.
5. Arruda LK, Sole D, Baena-Cagnani CE, Naspitz CK (2005). Risk factors for asthma and atopy. *Curr Opin Allergy Clin Immunol*, **5**(2):153–159.
6. Celedon JC, Litonjua AA, Ryan L, Platts-Mills T, Weiss ST, Gold DR (2002). Exposure to cat allergen, maternal history of asthma, and wheezing in first 5 years of life. *Lancet*, **360**(9335):781–782.
7. Peden DB (2005). The epidemiology and genetics of asthma risk associated with air pollution. *J Allergy Clin Immunol*, **115**(2):213–219.
8. McKeever TM, Britton J (2004). Diet and asthma. *Am J Respir Crit Care Med*, **170**(7):725–729.
9. Ford ES (2005). The epidemiology of obesity and asthma. *J Allergy Clin Immunol*, **115**(5):897–909.
10. Strachan DP (1989). Hay fever, hygiene and household size. *Br Med J*, **299**:1259–1260.
11. Ramsay C, Celedon J (2005). The hygiene hypothesis and asthma. *Curr Opin Pulm Med*, **11**:14–20.
12. Matricardi PM, Rosmini F, Ferrigno L, Nisini R, Rapicetta M, Chionne P, Stroffolini T, Pasquini P, D'Amelio R (1997). Cross sectional retrospective study of prevalence of atopy among Italian military students with antibodies against hepatitis A virus. *Br Med J*, **314**(7086):999–1003.
13. Peisong G, Yamasaki A, Mao XQ, Enomoto T, Feng Z, Gloria-Bottini F, Bottini E, Shirakawa T, Sun D, Hopkin JM (2004). An asthma-associated genetic variant of STAT6 predicts low burden of ascaris worm infestation. *Genes Immun*, **5**(1):58–62.

14. Heymann PW, Platts-Mills TA, Johnston SL (2005). Role of viral infections, atopy and antiviral immunity in the etiology of wheezing exacerbations among children and young adults. *Pediatr Infect Dis J,* **24**(11 Suppl): S217–222, discussion S220–221.

15. Hoffjan S, Nicolae D, Ostrovnaya I, Roberg K, Evans M, Mirel DB, Steiner L, Walker K, Shult P, Gangnon RE, Gern JE, Martinez FD, Lemanske RF, Ober C (2005). Gene-environment interaction effects on the development of immune responses in the 1st year of life. *Am J Hum Genet,* **76**(4):696–704.

Chapter 5

Common Precipitants of Asthma Exacerbations

Nikolaos G Papadopoulos and Chrysanthi L Skevaki

Introduction

Asthma exacerbations present with an increase in related signs and symptoms, which are unresponsive to the patient's routine medication and additional β_2-agonist therapy[1]. Such exacerbations may have either a rapid or gradual onset and are classified as mild, moderate or severe according to the severity of associated manifestations. Severity is assessed based on a number of parameters such as breathlessness, respiratory rate, accessory muscles and suprasternal retractions, degree of wheezing, peak expiratory flow (PEF) after initial bronchodilator and more (*Table 5.1*). The risk of developing severe exacerbations seems to be inconsistently related to the symptom severity of asthma.

As asthma prevalence is increasing in many countries, exacerbations are a major cause of morbidity and mortality, and still represent a challenge for the physician in terms of effective management. Indeed, asthma exacerbations, particularly severe ones, are a major cause of work and school day loss, sleep impairment, restricted activities, physician and accident and emergency visits, hospitalizations and the consequent increase in healthcare costs (*Table 5.2*).

A variety of factors have been associated with episodic worsening of asthma[2]. Such triggers act by aggravating lung inflammation and/or inducing acute bronchoconstriction.

Respiratory virus infection

Respiratory viruses are well-established causes of the majority of asthma exacerbations both in children and adults[3] (**5.1, 5.2**). Epidemics of exacerbations among asthmatic children are observed every September, coinciding with school return and peaks of respiratory tract infections[4]. The verification of this association followed the advent of the polymerase chain reaction (PCR), which allowed for sensitive respiratory virus detection (**5.3**). Indeed, application of PCR in a variety of epidemiological studies has confirmed a temporal association between viral detection peaks in the community and incidence of acute asthma attacks as well as asthma-related hospital admissions and mortality (**5.4**). Respiratory viruses have been isolated in up to 85% of asthma exacerbations in children and up to 60% in adults, the highest rates obtained in more recent, prospective studies using PCR.

The organisms most frequently involved in asthma exacerbations both in children and adults include rhinoviruses (RV), coronaviruses (**5.5**), influenza (IFV) and parainfluenza viruses (PIV) and respiratory syncytial virus (RSV), while adeno-, entero-viruses and human metapneumovirus are present at lower rates. Viral-induced exacerbations are most commonly slow in onset, typically following a common cold, and manifest with gradual increases in frequency and severity of cough and wheeze over a few days.

The prevailing agents are human rhinoviruses, which although classically considered as exclusively upper respiratory pathogens have now been shown to reach the lower airways and infect bronchial epithelial cells (**5.6**). Bronchial epithelial involvement is also a major feature of infection with other respiratory viruses such as IFV and RSV, resulting in cell death and local inflammation. Cellular debris, mucus and inflammatory cells aggregate in the airways producing significant narrowing, which resolves slowly due to the accompanying ciliary dysfunction. Peribronchial and submucosal oedema further aggravate this phenomenon. Loss of epithelial substances such as epithelium-derived relaxant factor and neutral endopeptidase may lead to decreased control over smooth muscle tone. Furthermore, epithelial cell death and defective ciliary clearance may result in enhanced

Table 5.1 Classification of asthma exacerbations according to severity*. Exacerbations are classified based on the presence of several (but not necessarily all) of the listed variables

Variable	Mild	Moderate	Severe	High risk of respiratory arrest
Breathlessness	On walking	On talking	At rest	
Ability to talk	Sentences	Phrases	Words	
State of alertness	Agitation possible	Agitation probable	Agitation probable	Drowsy/confused
Tachypnoea	Present	Present	Exaggerated	
Suprasternal and accessory muscle retraction	Usually not present	Present	Present	Paradoxical breathing
Wheezing	Moderate	Intense	Intense	Absent
Pulse rate	<100	100–120	>120	<60
Pulsus paradoxus	Absent	Possible	Probable	Absent when respiratory muscles are fatigued
PEF after initial bronchodilator (% of predicted or % of personal best)	>80%	60–80%	<60%	
PaO_2 (on air) and/or $PaCO_2$	Normal <45 mmHg	>60 mmHg <45 mmHg	<60 mmHg >45 mmHg	
SaO_2% (on air)	>95%	91–95%	<90%	

**Global Strategy for Asthma Management and Prevention*. National Institutes of Health Publication No 02-3659. Issued January, 1995 (updated 2002). Management Segment (Chapter 7): updated 2004 from the 2003 document.

permeability of allergens and irritants, augmenting allergen-induced inflammation (**5.7**).

Airway epithelial cells produce a variety of proinflammatory mediators such as kinins and nitric oxide and along with alveolar macrophages are responsible for the production of several cytokines, including interferon (INF)-α, -β and -γ, interleukin (IL)-1β, IL-6, IL-11, granulocyte macrophage colony stimulating factor (GMCSF), tumour necrosis factor (TNF)-α and the chemokines IL-8, regulated on activation, normal T-cell expressed and secreted (RANTES) and macrophage inflammatory protein (MIP)-1α[5]. Consequently, the mucosa is infiltrated with T lymphocytes, eosinophils and neutrophils. Viral infection may enhance histamine release from basophils and mast cells, and induce mast cell and eosinophil proliferation. Interacting cascades from the complement, coagulation, fibrinolytic and kinin systems of the plasma may also augment the inflammatory response. On the transcriptional level, transcription factor nuclear factor (NF)-κB appears to mediate the induction of several cytokines by respiratory viruses.

The host systemic immune response can also significantly influence the outcome of a viral infection. Antiviral

Table 5.2 Annual impact of uncontrolled asthma in the USA. Direct and indirect healthcare expenditure attributable to asthma exacerbations is a considerable part of the general cost of asthma. Numbers of various associated events are shown

Direct costs

Emergency visits	2 000 000*
Hospitalizations	500 000[†]
Unscheduled medical visits	7 400 000*

Indirect costs

Missed school days	14 000 000[‡]
Missed working days	14 500 000[‡]
Days of restricted activity	100 000 000[¶]

*American Lung Association (2002). Epidemiology and Statistics Unit, Best Practices and Program Services. *Trends in Asthma Morbidity and Mortality*. American Lung Association.
[†]Centers for Disease Control and Prevention (1998). Surveillance for asthma: United States, 1960–1995. *MMWR CDC Surveillance Summaries*, **47**.
[‡]Centers for Disease Control and Prevention (2002). Surveillance for asthma: United States, 1980–1999. *MMWR* **51**(SS01):1–13.
[¶]National Heart, Lung and Blood Institute (1997). *Expert Panel Report 2: Guidelines for the Diagnosis and Management of Asthma*. NIH Publication 97-5051. NIH, Bethesda.

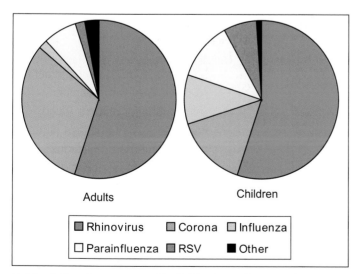

5.1 Isolation frequency of individual respiratory viruses in the context of acute asthma attacks. Rhinoviruses are responsible for the majority of viral-induced asthma exacerbations in both children and adults.

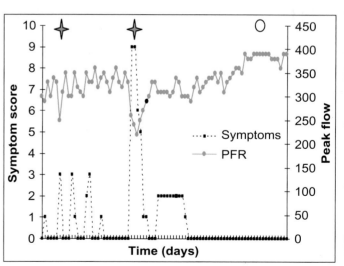

5.2 Daily symptom scores (dashed line) and peak flow measurements (solid line) of a child with asthma followed prospectively. The presence of respiratory viruses was assessed on three occasions: in the first two (star), a positive virus identification coincided with an increase in symptom scores and a drop in peak flow. In the third (open circle) no virus was present in agreement with the patient's report of no symptoms. NG Papadopoulos, unpublished data.

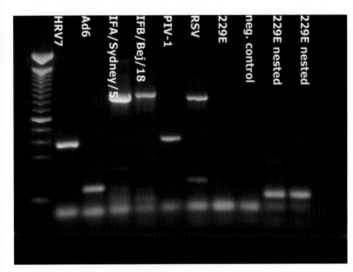

5.3 Gel electrophoresis of a multiplex polymerase chain reaction (PCR) simultaneously assessing the presence of various respiratory viruses in nasal secretions. Following the widespread use of similar PCR-based protocols it has been possible to assess the true impact of viral pathogens in a variety of respiratory diseases, including asthma exacerbations.

responses are usually dominated by T helper (Th)1 cytokines and interferon production. However, both Th1 and Th2 responses may be generated and, in atopic individuals, deviation towards Th2 cytokine production, which is considered crucial in the development of chronic allergic disease, may result in attenuated viral clearance and persistence of local inflammation.

Furthermore, neural mechanisms have been proposed to be involved, although data are less conclusive. Epithelial damage leaves underlying afferent nerve fibres exposed, possibly contributing to irritant susceptibility. Neuropeptide metabolism, dependent on epithelial cell integrity, may be compromised, as in the case of neutral endopeptidase 24–11, a major metabolizing enzyme of tachykinins. Viral infection also leads to alteration in neural receptor function with consequent neurogenic inflammation and altered smooth muscle tone. Dysfunctions of β-adrenergic receptors and increased cholinergic activity, resulting from inhibitory M2 receptor dysfunction have been shown in experimental models. Reflex bronchoconstriction and increased vascular permeability and airway secretions may result by this route (**5.8**).

Mechanical factors such as nasal obstruction resulting from upper respiratory tract infection may also contribute, since it leads to mouth breathing and therefore enhanced delivery of inhaled particles and colder, dryer air to the lungs. Recurrent viral-induced exacerbations may also possibly contribute to the progression of mild intermittent asthma to more severe and irreversible forms of the disease through remodelling of the airways.

Allergens

Atopic allergy is strongly associated with asthma. Therefore, it is reasonable that allergen sensitization and exposure have

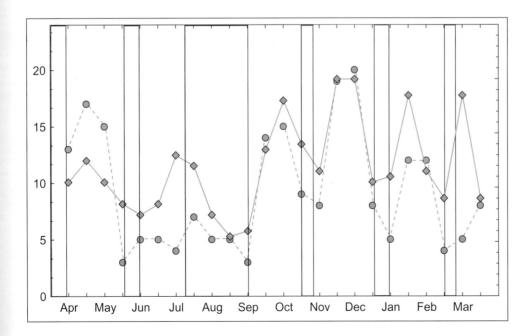

5.4 Correlation of virus isolation (dashed line) with hospital admissions for asthma (solid line) and school holidays (lineal areas). Asthma admissions coincide on most occasions with virus isolation peaks, which frequently follow the return to school. Redrawn with permission from Johnston SL *et al.* (1996). The relationship between upper respiratory infections and hospital admissions for asthma: a time-trend analysis. *Am J Respir Crit Care Med*, **154**(3 Pt 1):654–660.

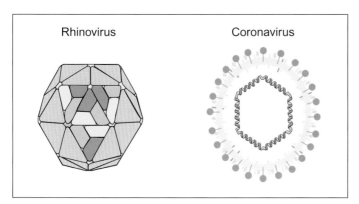

5.5 Diagrammatic representations of human rhinoviruses and coronaviruses, the agents most frequently isolated in common colds and acute asthma exacerbations. Together, these agents attribute for 70–80% of such events.

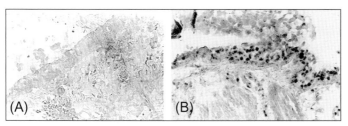

5.6 *In situ* hybridization for human rhinovirus RNA in bronchial biopsy sections from a human volunteer experimentally infected with the virus, before (**A**) and after (**B**) exposure. Positive signal, viewed as black dots, is obvious within epithelial cells after exposure. Reprinted with permission from Papadopoulos NG *et al.* (2000). Rhinoviruses infect the lower airways. *J Infect Dis*, **181**(6):1875–1884.

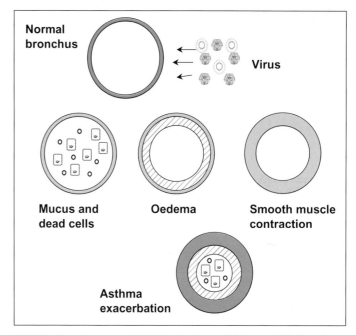

5.7 Mechanisms contributing to bronchial constriction in asthma exacerbations. The virus or other inducing factor may lead to mucus production, shedding of dead cells into the lumen, peribronchial and submucosal oedema and smooth muscle contraction. Added together, these mechanisms lead to considerable bronchoconstriction and an exacerbation of asthma.

long been considered as major triggers of acute exacerbations[6]. Seasonal and occasional associations of allergen level changes with epidemic asthma exacerbations are well documented. In Barcelona, epidemics of asthma exacerbations occurred on days when soybeans were being unloaded at a specific silo without a filter. Small amounts of airborne allergens can precipitate acute asthma attacks; however this also depends upon individual degree of sensitivity. Asthma epidemics, documented in several occasions after storms, have been attributed to the release of increased numbers of allergenic particles in the air. Among outdoor allergens, pollens and fungi are the most frequently encountered. Pollen allergens derive from grass, trees, and other plants and may cause seasonal exacerbations of asthma, varying with geographical location (**5.9**).

Over the past few years, indoor allergens, including house dust mites, animal and cockroach allergens, fungi, moulds and yeasts, have dramatically increased in Western households. Dust mite (*Dermatophagoides*, *Euroglyphus* species and other) allergens represent the most common asthmagenic agents in house dust and may infest beddings, carpets, and soft furniture (see **4.9(A)**). Storage mites are found in stored food and hay. Mite faeces contain allergenic proteolytic enzymes, while the bodies contain additional allergens. Concentrations of mite allergens above $0.5\,\mu g/g$ of dust are considered able to induce asthma exacerbations. Cats, dogs and rodents, such as wild mice and rats, are sources of a variety of allergens that are present in their saliva, excreta and danders. Fel d1 constitutes the principal cat allergen and is an almost ubiquitous, highly sensitizing and potent asthmagenic protein. Fewer people are sensitized to Can f1 and f2, the two most important dog allergens. *Alternaria*, *Penicillium*, *Aspergillus*, *Cladosporium* and *Candida* species, which belong to fungi, may also precipitate exacerbations and have occasionally been associated with severe exacerbations and death.

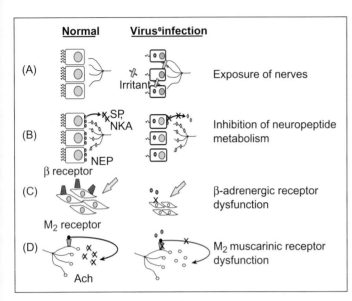

5.8 Proposed neural mechanisms of virus-mediated asthma exacerbations: epithelial destruction leads to (**A**) exposure of nerves to irritants or (**B**) inhibition of neuropeptide metabolism. Viruses may also attenuate the function of β-adrenergic receptors (**C**) and the M$_2$ inhibitory muscarinic receptor function (**D**). NEP, neutral endopeptidase; NKA, neurokinin A; SP, substance P; Ach, acteylcholine.

In human experimental models of allergen challenge (**5.10**), eosinophilic lung inflammation and airway hyper-responsiveness have been documented. However, real-life exposures to specific allergens are by rule at lower levels than those used in experimental settings; their effects are possibly mediated by repeated exposures, which may cause persistent inflammation and potentially structural changes, elements of airway remodelling.

Air pollution

The presence of high levels of irritants in the atmosphere has been proposed as a significant contributor in the development of asthma exacerbations[7]. Concentrations of pollutants in ambient air are determined by weather and geographical conditions. Susceptibility to air pollutants may also be determined by genetic factors such as those involved with antioxidant defences.

Industrial (sulphur dioxide particulate complex) and photochemical (ozone and nitrogen oxides) smog are the two main types of outdoor pollution[8]. Sulphur dioxide, which is a regulated pollutant in many countries can induce symptoms of acute asthma in afflicted individuals in a dose-dependent manner. Exposure levels to sulphur dioxide in the community are usually less than those known to evoke acute responses; however, some asthmatic subjects might experience associated symptoms at concentrations as low as 1 ppm. Diesel particles and nitrogen dioxide may account for the increased rate of exacerbations observed in populations living near roads with high-volume traffic. Ozone, aerosol sulphates, and aerosol hydrogen ions have been associated with airway inflammation, increased airway responsiveness

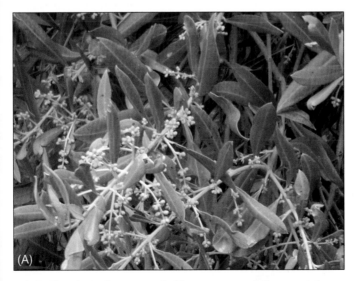
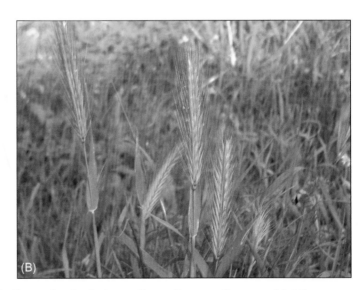

5.9 Pollinating olive trees (left) are some of the most frequent allergenic plants in southern Europe. Grasses (right) are more widespread and induce allergies worldwide.

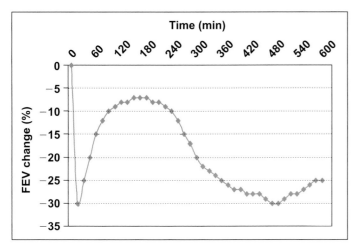

5.10 Changes in lung function, expressed as forced expiratory volume in 1 second (FEV_1), in a human experimental model of allergen exposure. The acute response results in a steep drop in FEV_1; the return to close-normal values is frequently followed by a late phase reaction 6–8 hours later.

and hospitalizations[9] (**5.11**). Exposure to increased levels of nitrogen dioxide has also been connected to increased asthma activity.

Indoor pollutants, including nitrogen dioxide, carbon monoxide and dioxide, sulphur dioxide and especially compounds of environmental tobacco smoke could be even more relevant[10]. Studies by the Environmental Protection Agency (EPA) report that levels of indoor pollutants tend to be two to five times (and in certain cases 100 times) higher than levels of outdoor pollutants. Cooking with natural gas or on wood, heating systems and tobacco exposure are only some of the sources. Burning tobacco produces thousands of harmful compounds such as tar particles, volatile hydrocarbons, carbon monoxide, and nitrogen oxides; environmental tobacco smoke (passive exposure) is associated with increased rates of exacerbations requiring medical attention (*Table 5.3*). Active smoking causes accelerated decline of lung function and more severe asthma in already asthmatic people. Household sprays and volatile organic compounds have also been associated with precipitation of acute asthma symptoms.

Given the diversity of air pollutants and the fact that they are present in mixtures of varying composition, the identification of a specific mechanism responsible for the induction of asthma attacks in susceptible individuals becomes a difficult task. Ozone and particulate matter may cause direct lung inflammation and oxidative stress due to a decrease in the glutathione/oxidized glutathione ratio. Carbon monoxide acts as a competitive inhibitor of oxygen transport via the formation of carboxyhaemoglobin. Moreover, other pollutants may modify enzymes, disrupt immune responses to allergens and facilitate coagulation.

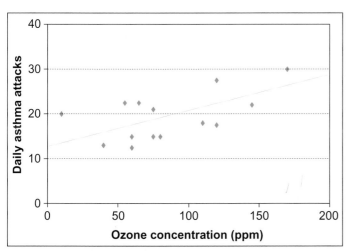

5.11 Asthma exacerbations increase in parallel to the increase in ozone concentrations. Data from Trasande L, Thurston GD (2005). The role of air pollution in asthma and other pediatric morbidities. *J Allergy Clin Immunol,* **115**(4):689–699.

Table 5.3 Constituents of environmental tobacco smoke. Tobacco smoke contains thousands of harmful compounds, some of which are listed below

Major	Minor
Tar particles	Aromatic substances
	• Fluoranthene
	• Benzopyrene
Carbon monoxide	N-nitrosamines
Nicotine	
Nitrogen monoxide	Radioactive isotopes
Volatile hydrocarbons	
• Ethane	
• Propane	
• Isopropane	

Exercise and hyperventilation

Exercise often causes reversible airflow limitation in asthmatic patients. Two major theories on its mechanism have been proposed: one attributes exercise-induced bronchoconstriction to the accompanying hyperventilation, which produces cooling and subsequent rewarming of the airway mucosa, while the other focuses on changes in the osmolarity of fluid lining the airway mucosa. Local release of mediators, such as histamine and leukotrienes from mast cells, precipitate acute bronchoconstriction. However, exercise is a rather specific stimulus for asthmatic patients, as it does not induce similar symptoms in either healthy individuals or patients with other respiratory diseases such as chronic bronchitis or cystic fibrosis. The majority of asthmatic patients, in some reports as many as 90%, experience worsening of their symptoms, ranging from mild discomfort to severe exacerbations, after varying degrees of exercise. In some patients, exercise can be the only inducer of symptoms. The term 'exercise-induced asthma' is widely used, although it may refer either to these patients, or to any patient experiencing exercise-induced bronchoconstriction. In any case, exercise-induced bronchoconstriction is responsible for the avoidance of physical activity by patients with asthma with unfavourable consequences for their health. Different sports are associated with variable degrees of asthmagenic capacity and this should be taken into account when consulting with patients intending to initiate or continue a sports activity (*Table 5.4*)[11]. On the

other hand, exercise-induced bronchoconstriction can also be a significant problem in elite athletes (**5.12**). However, exercise and hyperventilation do not seem to induce long-term changes in the airways and therefore are considered as 'inciters' of asthma.

Changes in weather

Asthma exacerbations have also been associated with extreme climatic conditions such as freezing temperatures and high humidity although this association remains controversial. Rainfalls, barometric pressure, and wind speed and direction represent other measures of local climatic

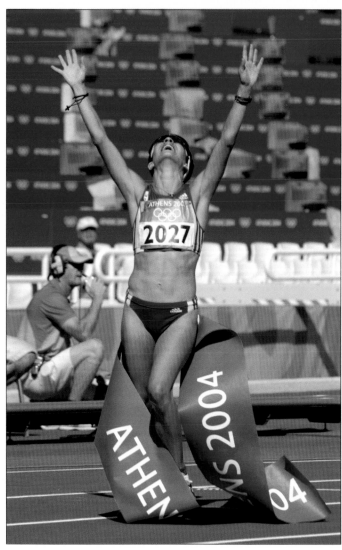

5.12 Asthma does not preclude elite athletes from becoming Olympic gold medallists. Reproduced with permission from A Tsoumeleka.

Table 5.4 Asthmagenic capacity of individual sports. Low/medium-risk sports are preferable for individuals intending to participate in sports activities and/or competition

High-risk	Medium-risk	Low-risk
• Running (long-distance)	• Basketball	• Running
• Cycling	• Volleyball	• Tennis
• Cross-country ski	• Football	• Fencing
• Ice hockey	• Rugby	• Gymnastics
• Ice skating	• Team sports	• Swimming
• Biathlon		• Waterpolo
		• Boxing
		• Alpine ski

conditions. Meteorological conditions may influence asthma activity indirectly by contributing to the clearance or accumulation of outdoor allergens. Indeed, thunderstorms, especially in late spring and summer, may cause epidemics of asthma exacerbations, possibly by increasing concentration of allergens in a shallow band of air at ground level. Moreover, the humidity preceding a thunderstorm may cause pollen grains to break up and release starch granules, which then circulate and precipitate their effects[12].

Occupational factors

Work-related asthma exacerbations are not rare, resulting from occupational exposure to irritants to which people are already sensitized (*Table 5.5*). Such sensitizers are classified in low and high molecular weight groups; the latter act in the same way as allergens in terms of inducing airway hyperresponsiveness, whereas the former's mode of action is less clear.

Foods, additives and drugs

Allergy to foods or additives has been implicated in the aggravation of asthma symptoms in some patients. However, although wheezing is one of the presenting symptoms of food-induced anaphylaxis, it is infrequently an isolated event. Food preservatives and other additives, such as those in wine, containing metabisulphite, may be a significant source of sulphur dioxide.

Table 5.5 Occupational allergens*. Numerous chemical substances are capable of precipitating acute asthma attacks in already sensitized people in the context of occupational exposure

Group of agents	Occupation
Isocyanates	Spray painter, foundry, plastics, rubber manufacturing, varnish, mold makers
Anhydrides	Plastics, epoxy resins and adhesives, polyester resin production
Amines	Spray painter, fur dyeing, cleaning products, welding, chemist, photography, lacquering
Metals (e.g. aluminum, tungsten, cobalt, zinc)	Grinder, platinum refinery, tanning, paints, metal plating, polishers
Drugs	Pharmaceutical company, healthcare workers
Plastics	Welders, meat wrappers
Dyes	Hairdressing, carmine extraction, food industry, photography
Animals	Agricultural, greenhouse workers
Insects	Food industry, laboratory workers, fish-feeders, silkworkers, mushroom workers, cleaners, millworkers, museum personnel
Fish and shellfish	Food industry, pearl industry tanners
Animal products	Food industry, laboratory workers, farmers, breeders
Plants and flours	Carpenters, food industry, floral worker, pharmacist, agriculture, gardeners, bakers
Woods	Sawmill, furniture, welders
Microorganisms	Bakers, carpenters, laboratory workers, cleaners, farmers
Enzymes	Bakers, laboratory workers, detergent industry, wood industry, food industry

*European Academy of Allergology and Clinical Immunology website: http://www.eaaci.net

On the other hand, dietary factors have been associated with increased asthma activity[13]. The Western diet, including consumption of highly processed foods, low vitamin and essential fatty acid intake seems to increase symptom rates, including exacerbations, in asthmatic people. Increased consumption of salt, alcohol and bioactive amines such as tyramine and histamine may also play a role. Moreover, obesity is associated with enhanced asthma morbidity and accelerated worsening of lung function.

Non-steroidal anti-inflammatory drugs (NSAIDs) precipitate asthma attacks, which are often dangerous, in about 10% of adult people with asthma. Aspirin-induced exacerbations are most probably due to overproduction of leukotriene C4. Paracetamol (acetaminophen) decreases lung glutathione levels and may result in increased oxidative injury and bronchospasm. β-blockers, heroin and many other drugs have also been implicated in asthma exacerbations (*Table 5.6*).

Endocrine factors

Worsening of asthma symptoms is occasionally observed in relation to menses or premenstrually. Furthermore, the

---

Table 5.6 Drugs associated with bronchoconstriction (asthma exacerbations)*

- NSAIDs: acetylsalicylic acid and others
- Steroids : hydrocortisone
- Antimicrobial agents: nitrofurantoin (acute)
- Antineoplastic: vinblastine/mitomycin
- Adrenergic agents: β-blockers
- Drugs of abuse : cocaine, heroin
- Other: contrast agents, nebulized drugs, IL-2
- Propafenone
- Protamine
- Dipyridamole

Global Strategy for Asthma Management and Prevention. National Institutes of Health Publication No 02-3659. Issued January, 1995 (updated 2002). Management Segment (Chapter 7): Updated 2004 from the 2003 document.

---

incidence of asthma exacerbations increases during pregnancy in one-third of cases, with consequent poor outcomes such as low birth weight, intrauterine growth restriction and pre-term delivery[14]. Thyrotoxicosis may also result in more frequent and more severe asthma attacks. Reactive oxygen species may be a contributory factor in exacerbating wheezing in this group of patients.

Stress – extreme emotional expression

Asthmatic people may experience exacerbations of their disease under psychological stress[15]. Extreme emotional expressions such as laughing or crying are usually accompanied by the increased general autonomic lability, the hyperventilation and hypocapnia and the resultant bronchoconstriction. Chronic stress induced by negative life events, a repressive coping style, as well as panic disorder also increase asthma morbidity in susceptible individuals.

Other

Bacterial pathogens are less common triggers of asthma exacerbations. Rhinitis, sinusitis, and polyposis have been implicated in the pathogenesis of exacerbations but evidence suggests indirect associations. It is more likely that such conditions rather represent a continuum of the same disorder, involving airway inflammation. Similarly, gastro-oesophageal reflux (GOR) has been suggested to precipitate acute asthma symptoms through vagally mediated and local axonal reflexes, heightened bronchial reactivity, and microaspiration, all resulting in neurogenic inflammation and acid-induced bronchoconstriction. Whether therapy of GOR improves asthma-associated symptoms in asthmatic people with GER remains controversial.

Synergy

Asthma exacerbations often occur as the result of interaction between several factors. The combination of viral infections with exposure to specific allergens in already sensitized asthmatic individuals act synergistically and may result in asthma exacerbations requiring hospitalization. Respiratory viral infections may facilitate penetration of allergens to airway submucosa due to the virally mediated epithelial destruction. Allergen-induced inflammation may increase by simultaneous exposure to air pollutants. Diesel particles have been shown to absorb pollen allergens on their surface and consequently deposit them on airway mucosa, enhancing their antigenicity. Acute concurrent exposure to allergen and cigarette smoke may cause enhanced airway responsiveness in sensitized patients. Air pollutants such as NO_2 may also interact with respiratory viral infections as well as occupational sensitizers and precipitate severe asthma exacerbations. Exercise may further complicate the effect of other factors.

References

1. *Global Strategy for Asthma Management and Prevention.* National Institutes of Health Publication No 02-3659. Issued January, 1995 (updated 2002). Management Segment (Chapter 7): Updated 2004 from the 2003 document.
2. Lemanske RF Jr, Busse WW (2006). 6. Asthma: Factors underlying inception, exacerbation, and disease progression. *J Allergy Clin Immunol*, **117**(2 Suppl Mini-Primer):S456–461.
3. Psarras S, Papadopoulos NG (2003). Respiratory virus infection of the lower airways and the induction of acute asthma exacerbation. In: *Respiratory Infections in Asthma and Allergy.* Johnston SL, Papadopoulos NG (eds). Marcel Dekker, New York.
4. Johnston NW, Johnston SL, Norman GR, Dai J, Sears MR (2006). The September epidemic of asthma hospitalization: school children as disease vectors. *J Allergy Clin Immunol*, **17**(3):557–562.
5. Papadopoulos NG, Papi A, Psarras S, Johnston SL (2004). Mechanisms of rhinovirus-induced asthma. *Paediatr Respir Rev*, **5**(3):255–260.
6. Murray CS, Poletti G, Kebadze T, Morris J, Woodcock A, Johnston SL, Custovic A (2005). A study of modifiable risk factors for asthma exacerbations: virus infection and allergen exposure increase the risk of asthma hospitalization in children. *Thorax*, **61**:367–368.
7. D'Amato G, Liccardi G, D'Amato M, Holgate S (2005). Environmental risk factors and allergic bronchial asthma. *Clin Exp Allergy*, **35**(9):1113–1124.
8. Atkinson RW, Strachan DP (2004). Role of outdoor aeroallergens in asthma exacerbations: epidemiological evidence. *Thorax*, **59**:277–278.
9. Chilmonczyk BA, Salmun LM, Megathlin KN, Neveux LM, Palomaki GE, Knight GJ, Pulkkinen AJ, Haddow JE (1993). Association between exposure to environmental tobacco smoke and exacerbations of asthma in children. *N Engl J Med*, **328**(23):1665–1669.
10. Rabinovitch N, Zhang L, Murphy JR, Vedal S, Dutton SJ, Gelfand EW (2004). Effects of wintertime ambient air pollutants on asthma exacerbations in urban minority children with moderate to severe disease. *J Allergy Clin Immunol*, **114**(5):1131–1137.
11. DiDario AG, Becker JM. Asthma, sports, and death (2005). *Allergy Asthma Proc*, **26**(5):341–344.
12. Marks GB, Colquhoun JR, Girgis ST, Koski MH, Treloar AB, Hansen P, Downs SH, Car NG (2001). Thunderstorm outflows preceding epidemics of asthma during spring and summer. *Thorax*, **56**(6):468–471.
13. James JM. Respiratory manifestations of food allergy (2003). *Pediatrics*, **111**(6 Pt 3):1625–1630.
14. Murphy VE, Clifton VL, Gibson PG (2006). Asthma exacerbations during pregnancy: incidence and association with adverse pregnancy outcomes. *Thorax*, **61**(2):169–176.
15. Sandberg S, Jarvenpaa S, Penttinen A, Paton JY, McCann DC (2004). Asthma exacerbations in children immediately following stressful life events: a Cox's hierarchical regression. *Thorax*, **59**(12):1046–1051. Erratum in: *Thorax*, 2005;**60**(3):261.

Churg–Strauss Syndrome

Cesar Picado

Introduction

Churg–Strauss syndrome (CSS) was first described in 1951 by the pathologists Lotte Churg and Jacob Strauss as an allergic and granulomatous small-vessel vasculitis. The three main histological features described by these authors were:

- tissue eosinophilia
- necrotizing vasculitis
- extravascular granulomas.

Churg and Strauss considered that their patients' condition represented a distinct inflammatory vascular process and suggested the term 'allergic granulomatosis and angiitis'. Later 'Churg–Strauss syndrome' became the generally accepted title of this form of systemic vasculitis.

Aetiology

The cause of CSS is unknown, and few data are available regarding its pathogenesis. In the 1960s it was proposed that the CSS was the result of an immune complex deposition. Triggering factors such as vaccination and allergen desensitization were suspected to be contributory factors to the development of the syndrome. These findings suggested the theory that microbiological and/or allergens were inducing vascular injury in a way similar to hepatitis B associated vasculitis. However, epidemiological studies failed to demonstrate any association between vaccination and immunotherapy with CSS. Moreover, in the majority of CSS cases it was not possible to show immune protein deposition in the vascular walls.

A few years after their introduction in the treatment of asthma, antileukotriene drugs were associated with CSS development, a finding that suggested that the syndrome might be precipitated by an idiosyncratic reaction to the drugs. However, many of the reported cases were diagnosed following reduction in the dose of corticosteroid, suggesting that the reduced dose of systemic corticosteroid therapy was the factor that caused the 'unmasking' of CSS. Similar cases of 'unmasked CSS' have been reported in patients receiving inhaled corticosteroids.

The discovery of antineutrophilic cytoplasmic antibodies (ANCAs) and the finding of ANCA in 40–65% of patients with CSS has led to the speculation that these antibodies may contribute to the pathogenesis of the process. Using indirect immunofluorescence, two major patterns can be recognized:

- a diffuse cytoplasmic staining (C-ANCA)
- a perinuclear/nuclear staining (P-ANCA).

Most of C-ANCAs are directed against proteinase-3, whereas approximately 80% of P-ANCAs recognize myelperoxidase. C-ANCA is preferentially associated with Wegener's granulomatosis and P-ANCA with microscopic polyangiitis (MPA) and CSS. However, this pattern is not disease specific because 10–20% of patients with classical Wegener's granulomatosis show P-ANCA and a similar percentage with CSS or MPA have C-ANCA. With regard to the specific role of ANCAs, the general hypothesis is that the antibodies produce tissue damage via interactions with neutrophils and endothelial cells. The initial events in the process require priming of neutrophils by cytokines and other stimuli, leading to the expression of proteinase-3 and myeloperoxidase on the cells surface.

In T cells the CDP95/CD95 ligand system is a major pathway of apoptotic cell death and thus essential for prevention of lymphoproliferative disorders and for autoimmunity. The CD95 system, which consists of membrane-bound (CD95Tm) and soluble (CG95Sol) receptor isoforms generated by alternative splicing and their natural ligand, CD95L, hold a key position in the regulation of the immune response. CD95Tm transduces the apoptotic signal after CD95L binding. In contrast, soluble CD95 can prevent target cells from undergoing apoptosis by neutralizing CD95L. Overexpression of soluble CD95 associated with oligoclonal T cell expansion has recently been reported in CSS. It has been suggested that the clonal T cell expansion might represent autoaggressive T cell population and that high levels of soluble CD95 may protect them from apoptotic removal. Furthermore, soluble CD95 was identified as a survival factor for eosinophils preventing their apoptosis. These findings suggest that impairment of CD95 ligand-mediated apoptosis of lymphocytes and eosinophils may be involved in CSS.

Presentation

CSS occurs with equal frequency in both sexes and can present at any age, with the mean age of onset being 40 years. CSS can affect virtually any organ in the body. Rhinitis is the first symptom in 75% of patients and it is characterized by discharge from the nose, often watery, nasal congestion and anosmia. Asthma is the central feature of CSS and precedes the systemic manifestations in almost all cases. It has been reported that many patients progress through a process of increasingly severe asthma to a stage characterized by eosinophilic pulmonary or gastrointestinal infiltration, preceding the development of vasculitis. Seventy-five per cent of the patients have received oral glucocorticoids for asthma symptoms prior to the diagnosis of CSS. Severe asthma is usually associated with chronic rhinosinusitis and nasal polyps in 70% of patients (**6.1**). General symptoms are frequent, and associated with pulmonary infiltrates in 38–77% of the patients. Radiologically, pulmonary infiltrates are usually transient and patchy in appearance (**6.2, 6.3**). The infiltrates lack lobar or segmental distribution but may be symmetrical (**6.4, 6.5**). Pulmonary infiltrates rarely cavitate and clinically symptomatic pleural effusions occur occasionally.

Although respiratory symptoms are the most common presenting feature of CSS, the site of the vasculitis

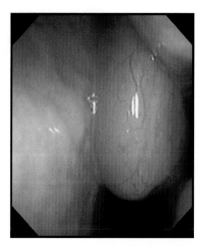

6.1 Nasal endoscopy in a patient with Churg–Strauss syndrome shows the presence of nasal polyps, which are similar in appearance and histological characteristics to common bilateral polyposis associated with asthma.

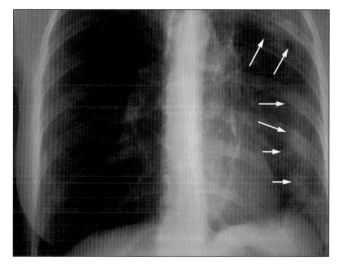

6.2 This chest X-ray was obtained from a 34-year-old woman admitted to the hospital with fever, asthma, diarrhoea, abdominal pain, paraesthaesias and weakness in the left lower extremity. Her white cell count was 15.600 with 34% eosinophils. The posteroanterior chest X-ray shows peripherally located airspace consolidations (arrows). Neurophysiological studies showed multiple mononeuropathies in the peroneal and femoral nerves. Test for antineutrophilic cytoplasmic antibodies (ANCAs) was positive with a typical perinuclear pattern of staining that was confirmed by enzyme immunoassay. The final diagnosis was Churg–Strauss syndrome.

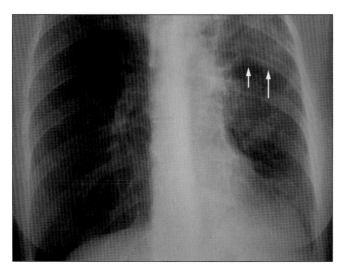

6.3 Posterior chest X-ray obtained 5 days after the one shown in **6.2**. The airspace opacities localized in the lower left lobe have almost disappeared whereas the opacity in the upper left lobe has enlarged. This is a typical characteristic of pulmonary infiltrates in Churg–Strauss that are usually transient, and patchy in appearance.

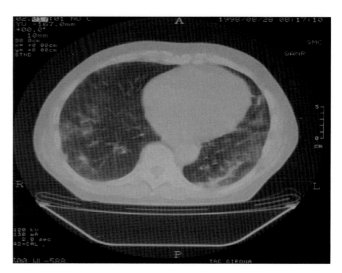

6.5 Lung computed tomography (CT) scan from the same patient as in **6.4**. The scan demonstrates areas of airspace consolidation in the periphery of both lungs that contrast with the opacities detected in the chest X-ray localized in the lower lobes and apparently less generalized than those detected with the CT scan. This discrepancy between the X-ray and CT occurs frequently.

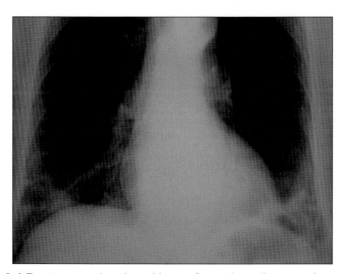

6.4 Posteroanterior chest X-ray of a patient diagnosed as having Churg–Strauss showing multiple zones of airspace consolidation in the lower lobes.

process is often outside the lungs, most commonly involving peripheral nervous system, skin, gastrointestinal tract, heart and kidney. Peripheral neuropathy, usually mononeuritis multiplex, is common (64–75%) in patients with CSS. When mononeuritis multiplex is seen in a patient with asthma and eosinophilia, the diagnosis of CSS is almost certain (**6.6**). Central nervous system involvement

is less frequent and may include palsies of the cranial nerves, convulsions, cerebral infarction or haemorrhage and coma.

Cutaneous lesions in the form of livedo reticularis, erythematous papules (**6.7**, **6.8**), palpable purpura (**6.9**, **6.10**), and subcutaneous nodules are seen in 40–70% of patients. Gastrointestinal involvement is frequent (37–62%). Abdominal pain is the most common clinical presentation and may be caused by vasculitis or eosinophilic gastroenteritis. Eosinophilic gastroenteritis may be followed by intestinal perforation. Eosinophilic ascites, pancreatitis and bloody diarrhoea also have been reported. These complications are predictive of a poor outlook in CSS patients.

Cardiac involvement is common, with pericarditis in 23% of the patients and eosinophilic endomyocarditis in 13%. Clinically, cardiac manifestations include congestive heart failure, pericarditis and dysrhythmias. Cardiac involvement has significant impact on patient morbidity and mortality, accounting for 20% of deaths seen with this disease.

Microscopic haematuria (68%) and proteinuria (63%) have been reported in CSS patients. Renal biopsy frequently shows focal segmental necrotizing glomerulonephritis (**6.11**) but unlike other necrotizing vasculitides, renal failure is rare.

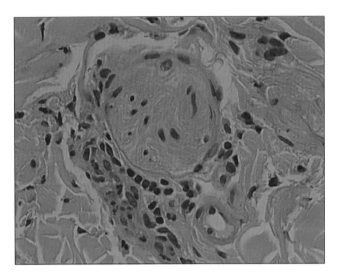

6.6 Skin biopsy disclosing a peripheral nerve with an eosinophilic infiltration (same patient as in **6.7**).

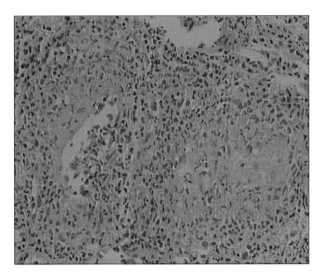

6.8 Skin biopsy from the same patient as in **6.7** shows a necrotizing vasculitis of small vessels with fibrinoid necrosis and eosinophilic infiltration.

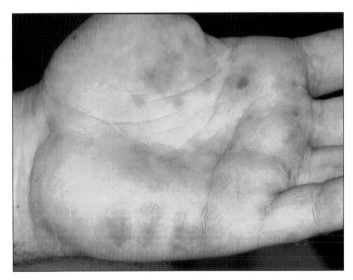

6.7 Erythematous papules in a 25-year-old man with history of rhinosinusitis, asthma and pulmonary infiltrates and marked eosinophilia in peripheral blood. He also complained of paraesthaesias and weakness in the right lower extremity. Test for antineutrophilic cytoplasmic antibodies (ANCAs) was positive with a typical perinuclear pattern of staining that was confirmed by enzyme immunoassay.

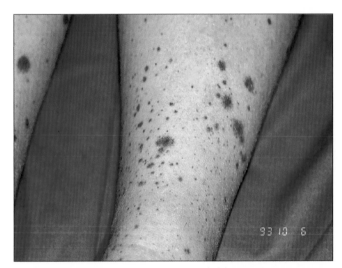

6.9 Purpura of the legs of a 45-year-old woman with asthma, pulmonary infiltrates, marked eosinophilia in peripheral blood and abdominal pain. Palpable purpura of the lower extremities is the most common lesion encountered in Churg–Strauss syndrome (CSS). Subcutaneous nodules of the limbs and scalp are also frequently seen in these patients. Although suggestive, these lesions are not pathognomonic, and do not distinguish CSS from other vasculitis.

Diagnosis

Diagnosis of CSS should be considered when a previously healthy individual presents with adult-onset persistent symptoms of rhinosinusitis associated with asthma followed by systemic symptoms (fever, weight loss), raised peripheral blood eosinophil count, fleeting pulmonary infiltrates and extrathoracic manifestations (gastrointestinal, cutaneous, nervous, cardiac or renal).

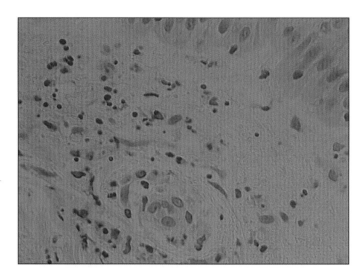

6.10 Skin biopsy from the patient with purpuric lesion (**6.9**) shows an apparently non-destructive eosinophilic infiltration of the walls of the small vessels.

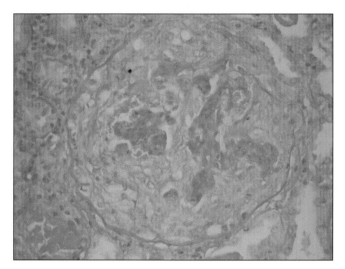

6.11 Renal biopsy frequently shows focal segmental necrotizing extracapillary glomerulonephritis in patients with Churg–Strauss syndrome (CSS). Renal involvement is present in 15–50% of the CSS patients but unlike other necrotizing vasculitis, renal failure is rare.

The investigation of a patient with suspected CSS involves exclusion of the known causes of eosinophilic pneumonia including parasitic infestations, allergic bronchopulmonary aspergillosis, chronic eosinophilic pneumonia and idiopathic hypereosinophilic syndrome. Typically chronic eosinophilic pneumonia is not associated with extrathoracic manifestations. Asthma and vasculitis are not present in patients with hypereosinophilic syndrome. Conventional diagnosis

of allergic bronchopulmonary aspergillosis is based on the demonstration of positive skin prick test and raised IgE to *Aspergillus*, positive precipitin test for *Aspergillus* and proximal bronchiectasis.

No laboratory finding is diagnostic for CSS. An elevated erythrocyte sedimentation rate and leucocytosis are common. One characteristic abnormality is peripheral eosinophilia. Approximately 90% of cases will exhibit an elevated eosinophil count at some point in the course of their disease. However, this eosinophilia may not be of long duration, and it will resolve rapidly once corticosteroid therapy has been instituted. Microscopic haematuria and proteinuria might indicate occult renal disease. Approximately 50% (higher in some series) of patients with CSS have ANCAs, most of them with perinuclear staining pattern (**6.12, 6.13**). Positive immunofluorescence assays must be confirmed by enzyme immunoassay; without this test isolated positive immunofluorescence is of limited utility.

An abnormal chest radiograph is usually found in 60–75% of patients with CSS. Infiltrates are often transient and peripherally distributed and can be associated with pleural effusion (25%) (**6.14**). This radiological pattern is

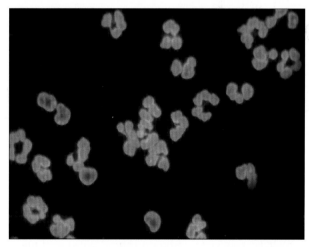

6.12 Immunofluorescence: P-antineutrophilic cytoplasmic antibody (P-ANCA) pattern. The perinuclear pattern reflects the presence of myeloperoxidase-ANCA in patients with vasculitis and is usually found in 40–60% of patients with CSS. This pattern is also frequently detected in other vasculitides such as microscopic polyangiitis and renal-limited vasculitis. In contrast, the P-ANCA pattern is rarely (10%) found in patients with Wegener's granulomatosis. The immunofluorescence assay was confirmed by enzyme immunoassay.

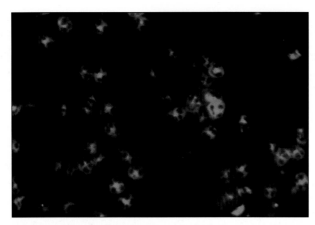

6.13 Immunofluorescence: C-antineutrophilic cytoplasmic antibody (C-ANCA) pattern. This pattern usually corresponds to the presence of proteinase-3 in vasculitis patients. The C-ANCA pattern is associated with Wegener's granulomatosis. The immunofluorescence assay was confirmed by enzyme immunoassay.

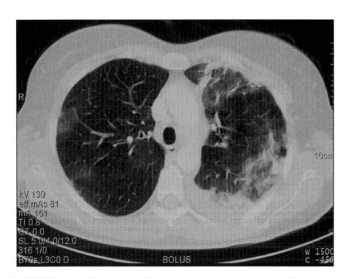

6.14 Thin section scan from the same patient as in **6.2** and **6.3** demonstrates extensive areas of airspace consolidation and ground glass attenuation. A small pleural effusion is also seen in the left hemithorax. Pleural effusions are relatively common (about 25%) and are usually small and manifest occasionally as pleuritic pain. The effusion is an exudate with high eosinophilia.

not specific to CSS, being seen in other conditions such as acute bronchopulmonary aspergillosis and chronic eosinophilic pneumonia. Sinusitis can be detected using computed tomography (CT) scans (**6.15**). Electrocardiogram and echocardiogram can confirm the presence of cardiac abnormalities.

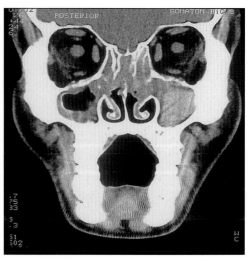

6.15 Coronal computed tomography scan of sinus of a patient with Churg–Strauss syndrome (CSS) demonstrates inflammatory mucosal thickening occluding the nasal cavity and paranasal sinuses. These abnormalities are usually present in 70% of CCS patients.

Ideally, biopsy of at least one involved organ should be done to confirm the presence of a necrotizing vasculitis accompanied by granulomas with eosinophilic necrosis (**6.16**). However, recent data indicate that characteristic pathological changes need not be present to establish the diagnosis of CSS. Some cases of CSS only show a simple eosinophilic infiltration without overt vasculitis (**6.17, 6.18**). In many cases an apparently non-destructive eosinophilic infiltration of vessel walls is the only relevant finding in biopsy materials. The widespread use of systemic corticosteroids in severe asthma often suppress the clinical manifestation of CSS, and this explains why changes in corticosteroid treatment may 'unmask' the disease. This type of '*formes frustes*' of CSS is usually diagnosed when corticosteroid-sparing therapies such as inhaled corticosteroids, antileukotrienes and chromones for asthma are introduced.

Treatment

The evolution of CSS changed dramatically with the introduction of corticosteroids, but prior to their use the prognosis of CSS was very poor. The recommended treatment is high-dose corticosteroids (60–80 mg of prednisone per day) for several weeks, followed by a schedule tapered according to the patient's clinical response. Intranasal and

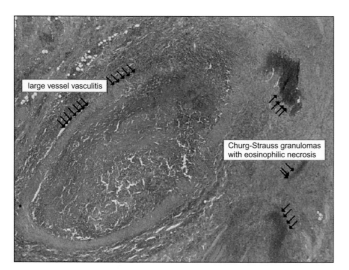

6.16 Biopsy showing the typical histological lesions in Churg–Strauss syndrome (CSS), composed of tissue eosinophilia, necrotizing vasculitis and extravascular granulomas. However, it is generally accepted that these pathological changes need not be present to establish the diagnosis of CSS. The initial description of histological lesions made by Churg and Strauss was based on a pathologic study of untreated patients who had died of the disease. Since then, many patients have been diagnosed as having CSS presenting without the classic histological findings. Such cases have been described as '*formes frustes*' of CSS and occur in patients who have been treated with corticosteroids for their asthma.

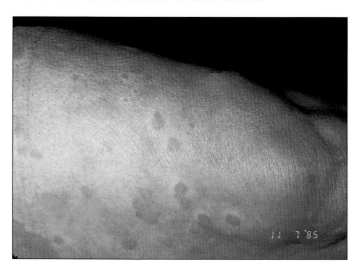

6.17 Urticarial vasculitis. In some Churg–Strauss patients dermal small-vessel vasculitis causes focal oedema resulting in urticaria. Urticaria associated with vasculitis persists longer than typical non-vasculitis urticaria and often evolves into purpuric lesions. Photo courtesy of Dr Raffaele Gianotti.

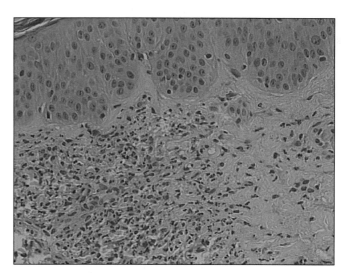

6.18 Skin biopsy in a patient with urticarial vasculitis. In many patients with Churg–Strauss syndrome diagnosed in early stages, tissue infiltration may take the form a simple eosinophilia in any organ as it was in this case.

inhaled corticosteroid therapy has been shown to be useful in reducing systemic corticosteroid requirements and should always be given to CSS patients with asthma and rhinosinusitis.

Oral cyclophosphamide (1–2 mg/kg/day) can be added on for those patients with limited response to corticosteroids and also to patients in whom CSS relapses when corticosteroids are discontinued. Combined therapy can also be indicated in patients with severe CSS characterized by substantial multi-organ involvement. Combined therapy appears to be more effective than single prednisone treatment in the prevention of CSS relapses. The reduced rate of relapse provided by combined therapy must be balanced against the increased risk of haemorrhagic cystitis, urological malignancy and serious infections. The risk of developing urological side effects appears to be related to the cumulative dose of cyclophosphamide. Strategies aimed at reducing the risk of chronic treatment with cyclophosphamide include the use of intravenous cyclophosphamide and the substitution of this drug by other immunosuppressive medication. The benefit of pulse intravenous cyclophosphamide ($0.6 \, \text{g/m}^2$ monthly) and oral treatment (2 mg/kg/day) was studied in a small group of CSS patients. Intravenous cyclophosphamide reduced the accumulative dose of the drug and was found to cause less side effects (alopecia, neutropenia, and haemorrhagic cystitis) than continuous oral therapy. Efficacy was comparable in both groups but unfortunately this conclusion is based on a study with a small number of patients.

Conclusions

CSS is distinct clinical disease characterized by a necrotizing vasculitis in patients with asthma and eosinophilia. Some CSS patients in whom the asthma is initially treated with systemic corticosteroids are not recognized until corticosteroids are tapered. Typically, asthma associated with rhinitis precedes the development of other manifestations. Mononeuritis multiplex is the most common form of neurological involvement. Typical dermatological findings include livedo reticularis, erythematous papules, palpable purpura and subcutaneous nodules. The most common gastrointestinal symptoms are abdominal pain and diarrhoea. Proteinuria is the most common manifestation of renal disease. One characteristic abnormality is fluctuating peripheral eosinophilia. Perinuclear antineutrophilic cytoplasmic antibodies occur in 40–60% of patients. Therapy begins with prednisone, and cyclophosphamide is added if the response is inadequate.

Further reading

Müschen M, Warskulat U, Perniok A, Even J, Moers C, Kismet B, Temizkan N, Simon D, Schneider M, Haussinger D (1999). Involvement of soluble CD95 in Churg-Strauss syndrome. *Am J Pathol*, **155**:915–925.

Noth I, Strek ME, Leff AR (2003). Churg–Strauss syndrome. *Lancet*, **361**:587–594.

Seo PH, Stone JH (2004). The antineutrophil cytoplasmic antibody-associated vasculitis. *Am J Med*, **117**:39–50.

Chapter 7

Pathology of Asthma

Wim Timens and Nick H T ten Hacken

Airway pathology in asthma: general features

Asthma is a chronic inflammatory condition of the lung, characterized in particular by inflammation of the large airways and, as has become clear, changes of the small airways and surrounding parenchyma. The pathological changes observed in these airways are due to short- and long-term effects of the presence of inflammatory cells, which in the long term lead to structural changes. These structural changes are often designated as 'remodelling', which comprises a change in size, volume or number of the resident cells or any of the structural components of a tissue. In the case of asthma, remodelling may be due to the (accumulated) direct effects of allergens or indirectly through injury and/or inflammation after contact with allergens. This also means that remodelling is accompanied by deleterious effects which in asthma in general are characterized by epithelial shedding, with loss of epithelial cells. Another characteristic feature is increase in thickness and change in constitution of the airway wall. In addition, mucosal changes with formation of mucus plugs in the airways also contribute to clinical manifestation of symptoms.

The characteristics of the pathological changes in the airways will be described and illustrated in the present chapter.

Normal airways

The normal airway is lined by an epithelial layer consisting of mainly ciliated cells and some goblet cells. The goblet cells, together with some mucus-producing glands in the airways, produce a thin layer of mucus which covers the cilia of the normal airway and functions as the first barrier to external deleterious effects. Just beneath the layer of ciliated and goblet cells, the epithelium further consists of basal cells which, in case of damage, are responsible for tissue repair and replacement of damaged parts of the epithelial cellular covering. The epithelium is attached to the reticular basement membrane (RBM), and directly beneath this area is the submucosa, composed of a loose extracellular matrix in which small vessels and nerves are present and occasional inflammatory cells can be observed. In the deeper parts of the submucosa, airway smooth muscle is present.

Pathogenesis of allergic airway inflammation

In allergic asthma the inflammatory pathological changes in the airways are the end result of a specific reaction to allergen exposure. Asthma is a disease which is the result of a pulmonary manifestation of a mixture of acute inflammation, mediated largely by type 1 hypersensitivity reactions and chronic inflammation. This is largely mediated by T cells, with mast cells, eosinophils and sometimes neutrophils being the major effector cells. Type 1 hypersensitivity reaction represents an abnormal tissue response to a certain antigen (which, because of this abnormal response, is termed 'allergen') in a predisposed individual. In a sensitized individual, exposure to this antigen would have led to the production and presence of a particular type of immunoglobulin, IgE. When such an individual is exposed to the allergen, the tissue response is a type 1 hypersensitivity reaction that starts rapidly (minutes) after interaction of the allergen with IgE, previously bound to high-affinity receptors for IgE on the surface of mast cells residing in the airway wall. Basophils closely resemble mast cells, including the high-affinity IgE receptors, but are present in only low numbers in the blood, and not normally in tissues. In case of inflammation these cells can be recruited from the circulation.

After exposure to allergen, often an early and a late phase response can be discerned. Patients can have both an early and a late response to direct exposure to an allergen or can show only an early phase reaction or a late phase reaction. Clinically, both phases are characterized by shortness of breath and wheezing. The early phase starts within minutes after allergen exposure and generally lasts 1–2 hours, after which, often with an interval with fewer symptoms, the late phase reaction can follow.

The allergen directly breaks down epithelial tight junctions, and activates epithelial cells and dendritic cells present in the epithelium. Subsequently, the classic early phase immunological reaction is supposed to be mainly the result of direct activation of mast cells as indicated above (**7.1**). The pathological changes initially observed have been chiefly associated with effects of primary mediators, mainly granular contents, such as histamine, present in mast cells (**7.2**), although recent results from studies with antileukotriene compounds suggest that leukotrienes likely play a more important role even in the early response. The same is likely to be true for prostaglandins. The late phase reaction is associated with activation of the specific immune system with predominant involvement of T helper (Th2)-type CD4 T cells, which activate and attract eosinophils (**7.1**). The time it would take for migration of CD4 T cells and eosinophils, together with time for formation of mast cell secondary mediators, such as prostaglandins, leukotrienes and platelet-activating factor (PAF), is supposed to be the main

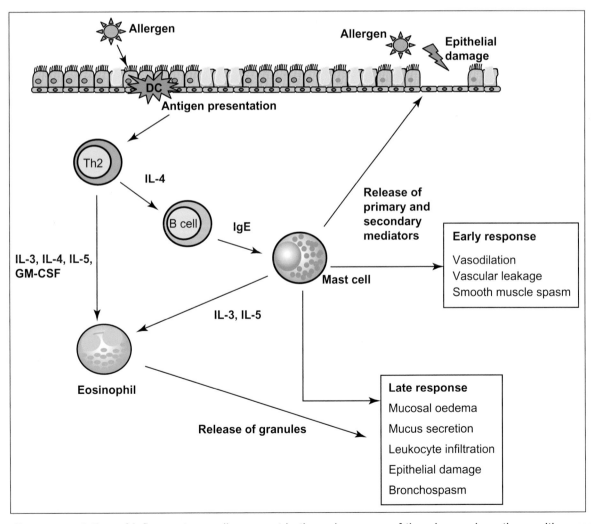

7.1 Schematic representation of inflammatory cells present in the submucosa of the airways in asthma with some of the main mediators produced by these cells. DC, dendritic cell; IL, interleukin.

explanation for the relatively late appearance of symptoms. The local changes in the airways in this late phase are mainly attributed to mediators produced by eosinophils (**7.3**) and secondary mediators produced by mast cells (**7.2**). Biopsy studies of patients with asthma, employing provocation with an allergen, have shown that already in an early phase a rather extensive infiltration of eosinophils and CD4 cells can be observed (**7.4** and **7.5**).

As described above, in addition to the direct effect of the allergen on local mast cells, the specific immune response is stimulated. The allergen stimulates epithelial cells to produce mediators that activate and recruit dendritic cells, Th2 cells and eosinophils. The allergen is presented by the dendritic cells to the Th2 cells and, at the same time, the dendritic cells are activated to produce more chemokines for these Th2 cells (see overview in **7.6**).

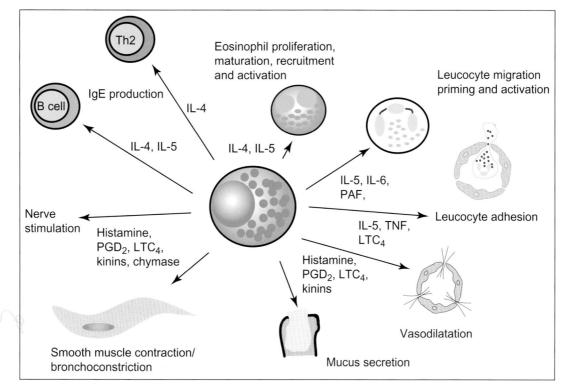

7.2 The main mediators produced by mast cells with indication of their most important effects. IL, interleukin; PGD$_2$, prostaglandin D$_2$, PAF, platelet-activating factor; TNF, tumour necrosis factor.

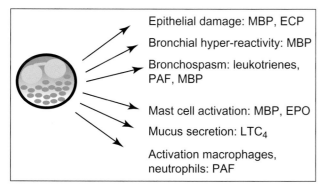

7.3 Effects of eosinophil activation with contributing mediators. MBP, major basic protein; ECP, eosinophil cationic protein; EPO, eosinophil peroxidase; PAF, platelet activating factor.

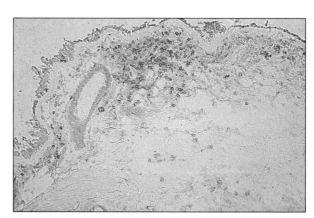

7.4 Immunostaining for CD4 at 3 hours after provocation with allergen: many CD4-positive (T helper) cells are already present in the early reaction.

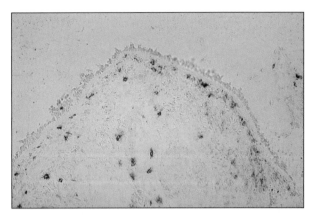

7.5 EG2 positive staining of eosinophils at 3 hours after provocation in an asthmatic airway: note already in this phase the presence of numerous eosinophils in the airway.

In the airways Th1 CD4 cells are also present that counteract many activities of Th2 cells and vice versa (*Table 7.1*). Because of the above described cascade of events after allergen exposure in asthma, an imbalance between Th1 and Th2 cells is established in favour of Th2 effects. More recently it has been suggested that Th2 effects as such might be inhibited by local presence of so-called regulatory T cells (Treg cells; *Table 7.2*), and it was speculated that insufficient inhibition by either natural Treg cells or adaptive Treg cells may play a role in the pathogenesis of asthma.

Role of nitric oxide and nitric oxide synthase in inflammation

Nitric oxide is a molecule that plays an important role in inflammation by its ability to contribute to the killing of tumour cells, viruses, bacteria and other microorganisms. To this end, the necessary high concentrations of nitric oxide are mainly the result of an increase of inducible nitric oxide synthase (iNOS) in inflammatory cells (see *Table 7.3* for overview of characteristics and **7.7** for a schematic overview of the role of nitric oxide synthases). In addition, nitric

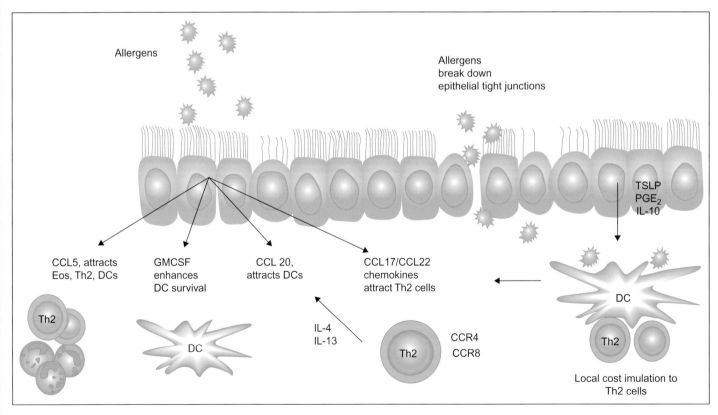

7.6 Interaction of epithelial dendritic cells (DCs) and T helper (Th)2 cells after allergen challenge. GMCSF, granulocyte macrophage colony stimulating factor; IL, interleukin; TSLP, thymic stromal lymphopoietic cytokine; PGE$_2$, prostaglandin E$_2$; Eos, eosinophils. Modified from van Rijt LS, Lambrecht BN (2005). Dendritic cells in asthma: a function beyond sensitization *Clin Exp Allergy*, **35**:1125–34.

Table 7.1 Characteristics of Th1 and Th2 cells

	Th1	Th2
Cytokines	• IL-2, IFN-γ • IL-3, GMCSF	• IL-4, IL-5, IL-10, IL-13 • IL-3, GMCSF
Main receptors	• IL-12Rβ, IL-18R • CXCR3, CCR5	• CCR4
Effector functions	• Macrophage activation • Complement-binding • Opsonization • Neutrophil activation	• Production of IgE • Production of neutralizing antibodies • Suppression of macrophage activation • Eosinophil activation, proliferation, maturation, recruitment

GMCSF, granulocyte macrophage colony stimulating factor; IL, interleukin; IFN, interferon; IgE, immunoglobulin E.

Table 7.2 Characteristics of regulatory T (Treg) cells

nTreg	aTreg: Th3	aTreg: Tr1
• T cell: T cell/APC contact • Generated in thymus • CD4+, CD25hi, CD45RO+, GITR+, CTLA4+, CD103+, Foxp3+ • Protect against autoimmunity • 5–10% of CD4+ T cells	• Soluble/membrane TGF-β • Generated in periphery (post-thymic) • Variable CD25 expression • Inhibit Th1 and Th2 responses	• Soluble IL-10 • Generated in periphery • (post-thymic) • Variable CD25 expression • Inhibit Th1 and Th2 responses

Major characteristics of subsets of CD4+ Treg cell bases on cell-surface markers, immunosuppressive cytokine secretion and suppressive action. nTreg, natural Treg; aTreg, adaptive Treg; Th, T helper cell; Tr1, T-regulatory cell type 1; APC, antigen-presenting cell, TGF, transforming growth factor; IL, interleukin. (From Van Oosterhout AJ, Bloksma N (2005). Regulatory T-lymphocytes in asthma. *Eur Resp J*, **26**:918–932.)

oxide as produced by constitutive NOS (cNOS) not only has a role in vascular relaxation in the lung, but also has airway relaxing characteristics with a direct relaxing effect on smooth muscle of the airways. The high concentration of nitric oxide and nitric oxide metabolites necessary for effective immune function can also have deleterious effects on local tissues.

As asthma is characterized by a chronic inflammatory process, it too involves positive and negative effects of nitric oxide. In the initial inflammatory changes in the airway, proinflammatory cytokines such as interferon-γ and tumour necrosis factor (TNF)-α and interleukin (IL)-1β lead to increased expression of iNOS in epithelial cells and macrophages. This leads to increased nitric oxide which in turn contributes to eosinophilic inflammation by chemotaxis of eosinophils and inhibition of apoptosis of eosinophils. In addition, the local high concentration of nitric oxide probably leads to local tissue damage supposedly mainly by peroxynitrite, a metabolite of nitric oxide. Another characteristic feature of nitric oxide is that it causes and amplifies an imbalance between Th1 and Th2 CD4 cells. In clinical practice, inhibitors of nitric oxide production have not demonstrated a recognizable effect in recent studies. There are indications that inhaled corticosteroid use may be effectively titrated on the basis of nitric oxide concentrations in exhaled air.

Table 7.3 Characteristics and effects of constitutional nitric oxide synthase (cNOS) and inducible NOS (iNOS)*

	cNOS	iNOS
Presence	Permanently present in the cells and the tissues that are able to produce cNOS	Absent under normal conditions, only developed under extreme conditions
Localization	• type I (or eNOS): endothelium, epithelium, smooth muscle • type III (or nNOS): non-adrenergic, non-cholinergic neural system (NANC)	Macrophages, monocytes, leukocytes, airway epithelium, endothelium
Stimulus	Acetylcholine, histamine, leukotrienes, bradykinin, ADP, ATP, VIP, PAF, substance P, calcium-ionophore	Endotoxin, LPS, proinflammatory cytokines such as IFN-γ, IL-1β, TNF-α, TNF-β
Production decreases by	Nitric oxide and smoking	Corticosteroids
Dependent on	Calcium and calmodulin	Transcription of DNA
Reaction time	Seconds up to minutes	Hours
Duration	Short	Long-lasting
Nitric oxide production	Pico molars	Nano molars
Nitric oxide effect	Physiological: neurotransmission, vasodilation, anti-thrombocyte aggregation, airway dilatation	Pathophysiological: tumour cell killing and antigen inactivation, cytotoxicity, dysregulation of cNOS-mediated effects

*cNOS may be inducible and iNOS can be constitutively present.
ADP, adenosine diphosphate; ATP, adenosine triphosphate; IFN, interferon; IL, interleukin; LPS, lipopolysaccharide; PAF, platelet activating factor; TNF, tumour necrosis factor; VIP, vasoactive intestinal polypeptide.
Modified from Ten Hacken NH *et al.* (1999). [Nitric oxide and asthma]. *Ned T Geneesk*, **143**:1606–1611 [Article in Dutch].

Pathology of allergic airway inflammation

Even in mild cases, asthma is a characterized as a chronic inflammation of the large and small airways and surrounding lung parenchyma (**7.8**). The cellular components of this inflammation consist of increased numbers of activated CD4 (lung Th) lymphocytes with associated eosinophilia. Within the CD4-positive T cells a predominance of the type 2 Th cytokines IL-4 and IL-5 together with increased presence of eosinophil chemoattractants including eotaxin and 'regulated on activation, normal T-cell expressed and secreted' (RANTES) is observed. This local cytokine microenvironment is supposed to be mainly responsible for the local tissue eosinophilia. Also an increase in mast cells is observed, in particular in association with airway smooth muscle. The persistence of inflammation in the asthmatic airways is likely to be not only because of the increased chemotaxis of Th2 cells and eosinophils but also because of the altered regulation of inflammatory cell survival by reduction of apoptosis. The number of apoptotic eosinophils as well as macrophages has been shown to be far fewer in people with asthma compared with chronic bronchitis.

The inflammatory changes in severe asthma are, in part, similar to more mild cases but, in addition, an inner wall neutrophilia and an increase in mast cells in the outer wall has been reported. In fatal asthma an increased number of CD8-positive cells has been observed, but these cells are also found in substantial numbers in mild asthma (**7.9**). Severe exacerbations of asthma are also characterized by an increase in the number of neutrophils, which can partly be explained by an increase in chemoattraction by locally produced neutrophil chemokines such as IL-8 (also designated

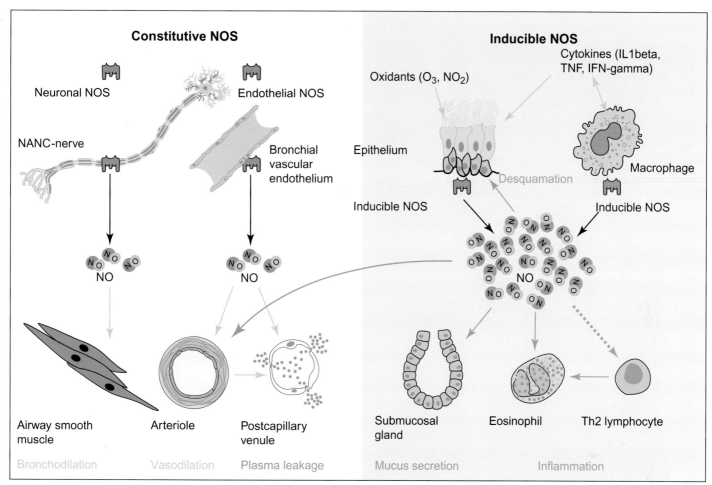

7.7 Schematic representation of role of nitric oxide (NO) synthases (NOS) in normal and pathological circumstances. IL, interleukin; IFN, interferon; TNF, tumour necrosis factor. Modified from Ten Hacken NH *et al.* (1999). [Nitric oxide and asthma]. *Ned T Geneesk*, **143**:1606–1611 [Article in Dutch].

as CXCL8) and CXCL5. These chemokines can be released by a large array of cells locally present in the airways, including epithelial cells and fibroblasts. The inflammatory changes in exacerbations therefore seem not to be specific but rather to represent the result of a general local activation of the innate immune defence system.

sticky mucus may lead to obstructive plugging in smaller airways with the collapse of lung areas. Besides mucus, these plugs contain cellular debris, inflammatory cells and their secretions, and shed epithelial cells. In mucus casts, and sometimes on histological examination, these constituents form so-called Curschmann's spirals.

Intraluminal obstruction in asthma

In asthma, the airways are filled to a variable extent with mucus of a tenacious structure (**7.10**). This is the result of increased mucus production by the epithelial goblet cells and hypertrophic submucosal glands stimulated by inflammatory mediators. In addition, neurogenic influences contribute to increased local mucus production. This overproduction of

Epithelial injury

As indicated above, local airway inflammation, with release of several deleterious mediators, and, in addition, the increased presence of nitric oxide may lead to local injury. In histological specimens from individuals with asthma, local damage and shedding of airway epithelium are often observed (**7.11**). In the copious mucus in the bronchial lumen, large

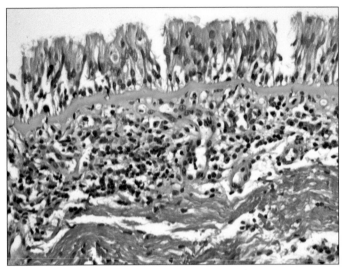

7.8 Inflammatory changes in the asthmatic airway: a mixed inflammatory infiltrate is seen in the submucosa with involvement of the epithelium. The inflammatory infiltrate is mainly composed of lymphocytes with eosinophils.

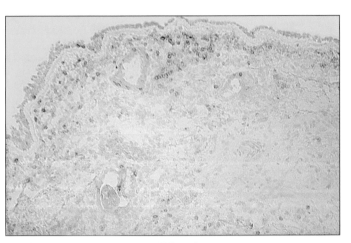

7.9 CD8-positive cells in mild asthma.

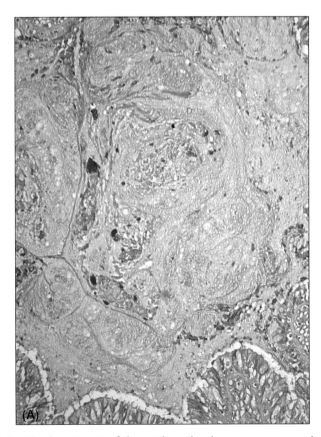

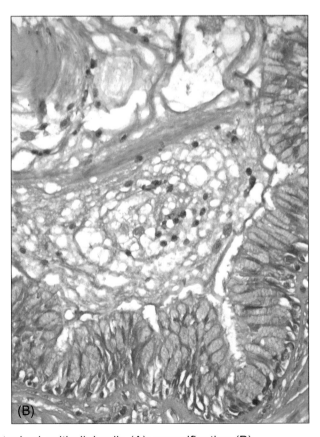

7.10 Luminal contents of the asthmatic airway: mucus and detached epithelial cells (A); magnification (B).

clusters of locally detached epithelial cells can be observed (also called Creola bodies when seen in sputum specimen). This detachment of epithelial cells seems to be the result of the above described damaging effect. This mostly concerns detachment of the suprabasal epithelial cells (**7.12**), whereas the basal cells mainly remain attached to the reticular basement membrane (RBM). This may be because the type of intercellular attachment is different from that involved in attachment of basal cells to the RBM, and that these intercellular attachments seem more vulnerable. Very often eosinophils and lymphocytes are seen quite near the area of detached epithelial cells (**7.13**) leading to the suggestion that mediators of eosinophilic granulocytes, in particular, play a role in this epithelial damage and loss of suprabasal epithelial cells. It is not quite certain whether this detachment of epithelium is actually an increased real damage or whether it represents an increased vulnerability in response to very mild physiological stimuli. The epithelium also plays an important role in remodelling of the underlying submucosa, and the mesenchymal cells such as fibroblasts present within this area (and vice versa). This complex mutual interaction

of epithelial and mesenchymal cells has been termed the epithelial–mesenchymal trophic unit. The most characteristic interactions are depicted in **7.14**.

Airway wall remodelling

The thickening of the airway wall in asthma is largely due to short- and long-term effects of ongoing inflammation. The short-term effects are vasodilatation and oedema, and hyper-reactivity or spasm of the airway smooth muscle. These effects cause stiffening of the airway wall with reduction of airway calibre. In addition, the above described epithelial changes, with damage and loss of epithelial cells, are part of the short-term remodelling events. A long-term effect observed in the epithelium is the relative increase in mucus-containing goblet cells (**7.15**), although this is a less pronounced feature than in chronic obstructive pulmonary disease.

Although not really a short-term effect, thickening of the basement membrane is observed in early stages of asthma, and even in mild cases (**7.16**), not only in the large but also in the smaller airways (**7.17**). As has become clear, this is not a thickening of the RBM but is a deposition of extracellular matrix proteins on the basal side of the RBM (**7.18**). How far this thickening contributes to airway obstruction is unclear. The thickness itself does not seem to be related to symptoms or severity of airflow limitation, but it is conceivable that it may be a constant factor in the airflow obstruction, with superimposed obstructive effects of actual inflammation, including increased smooth muscle volume and contraction.

The contribution of the increase of vessels in the airway to airway wall thickening is difficult to determine. Vasodilatation seen in a tissue section may lead to the impression that an increased proportion of the bronchial wall is occupied by vessels. Angiogenesis as a contributing factor has incidentally been reported in mild asthma but seems to be marked largely in severe corticosteroid-dependent asthma.

Increase in smooth muscle mass (**7.19**) is considered a consistent long-term feature of airway wall remodelling in asthma, although most studies have been performed in fatal asthma. This increase in smooth muscle volume is thought to be caused by hypertrophy and/or hyperplasia of smooth muscle fibres, but no definite conclusions can be draw as yet. With respect to these observations of smooth muscle changes it should be recognized that these are related to

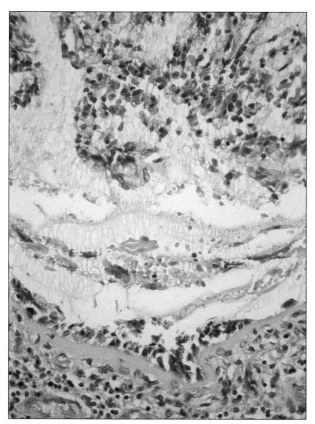

7.11 Mucus in asthmatic airway with extensive epithelial shedding.

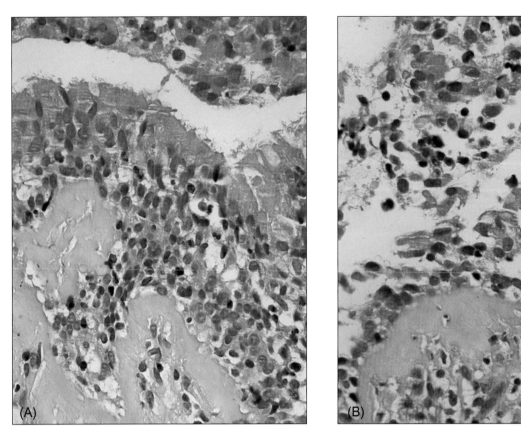

7.12 Biopsy of asthmatic airway with (A) beginning as well as (B) more advanced detachment of the epithelium due to local inflammation.

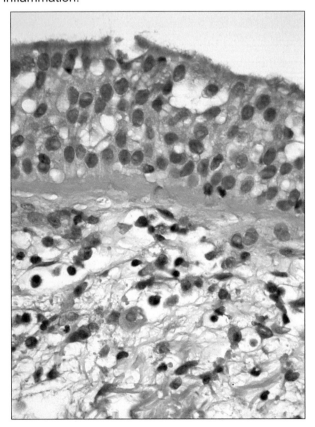

7.13 Partly damaged epithelial cells with eosinophils infiltrating the epithelium.

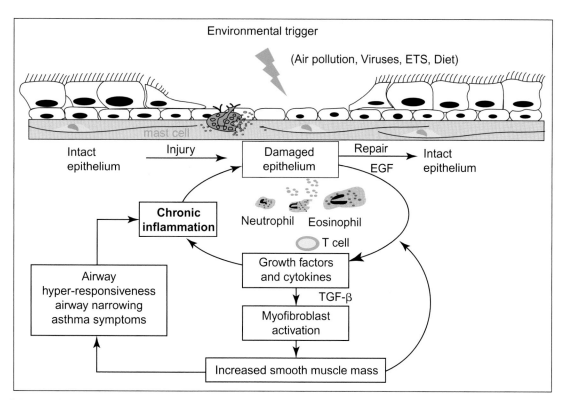

7.14 Model of the epithelial–mesenchymal trophic unit (EMTU) in chronic asthma indicating communication between the damaged epithelium and underlying fibroblasts and matrix, ultimately leading to remodelling. Cytokines generated as part of the inflammatory response interact with this unit influencing remodelling. EGF, epidermal growth factor; TGF, transforming growth factor. From: Holgate *et al.* (2004) *Proc Am Thorac Soc*, **1**(2):93–98.

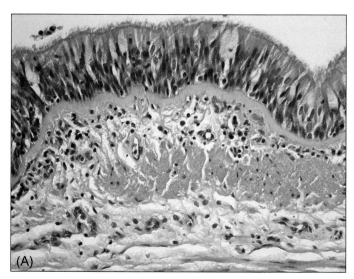

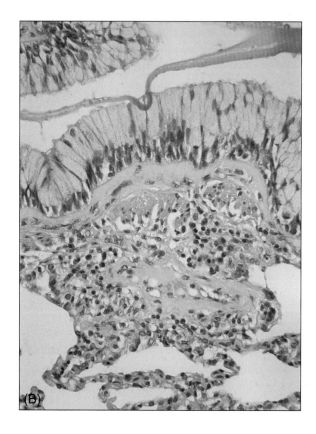

7.15 Asthmatic airway epithelium: increase in goblet cells varying from few (A) to many (B).

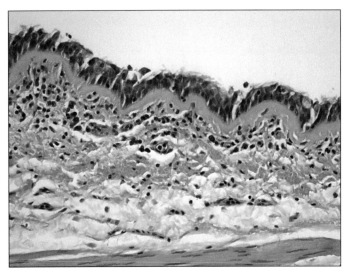

7.16 Thickened basement membrane in asthma: in the asthmatic airway the basement membrane is evenly thickened with clear eosinophilic staining.

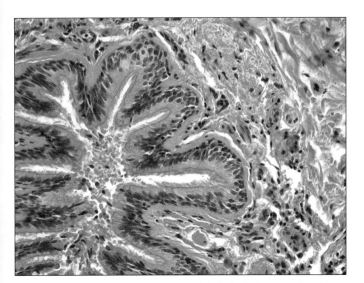

7.17 A small airway in asthma with little inflammation but clear thickening of basement membrane.

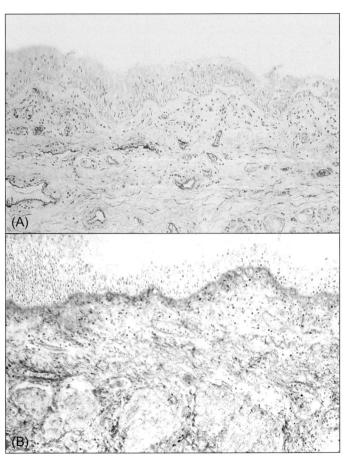

7.18 (**A**) Laminin staining showing staining of the true reticular basement membrane, whereas the matrix deposited at this site remains negative. (**B**) Collagen 1 immunostaining showing deposition of extracellular matrix at the basal side of the true reticular basement membrane.

airway diameter, and that it is thus very difficult to exclude a contribution of a state of increased contraction in lung resection specimen as used for most studies. Such increased contraction would in fact lead to an observation of temporary increase in muscle volume in an airway with temporarily decreased airway diameter.

Peribronchial pathology

Initially the inflammatory process in asthma was supposed to be present mainly in the submucosa of large airways, and observations with respect to adventitial and peribronchial inflammation mainly came from cases of fatal asthma. Most information on inflammation and other pathological changes in day-to-day asthma has come from biopsy studies that for a long time were limited to mucosal biopsies. Recently, studies have been performed on transbronchial biopsies that indicated that asthmatic inflammation is probably not confined to the bronchial submucosa but extends to the adventitia and peribronchial attachments (**7.20, 7.21**).

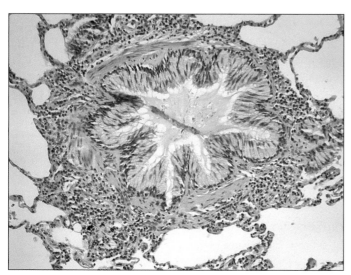

7.19 Cross-sectional view of severely contracted small airway in a 22-year-old woman with fatal asthma as a result of peanut allergy.

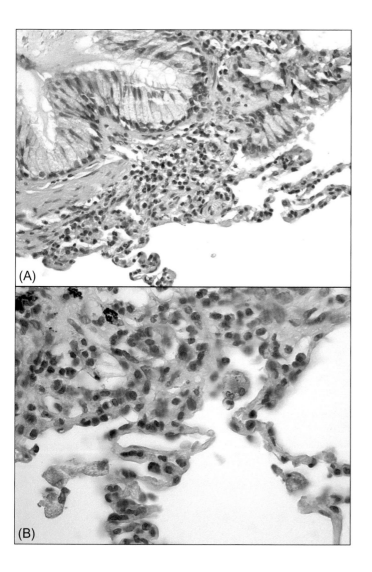

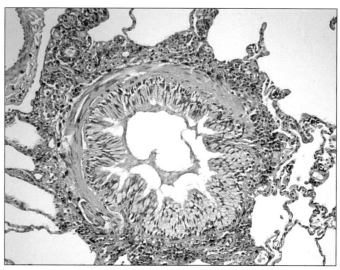

7.21 Asthmatic airway in fatal asthma: besides eosinophilic granulocytes (**7.19, 7.20**) there is an impressive increase of tryptase positive mast cells (dark brown; immunoperoxidase) in the adventitia.

Concluding remarks

Asthma is a common disease that can have considerable impact on daily life. Insight into the underlying pathological processes of the disease has contributed to development of therapeutic strategies and devices that have provided relief to most patients. Historically, the first valuable information with respect to pathology came from post-mortem studies of fatal and severe asthma. The broad introduction of flexible bronchoscopy some decades ago allowed great advances by enabling study of pathological changes in mucosal biopsies and broncho-alveolar lavage in asthmatic people with or without symptoms, during exacerbations and so on. Although still limited, recently transbronchial biopsies have also been undertaken in some centres. Since the introduction of flexible bronchoscopy, studies of pathology of asthma have allowed fine-tuning of therapy and development of more adequate and more convenient inhalation devices.

Further studies on and insight into the pathology of asthma, in conjunction with other important areas such as genetics (functional genomics and pharmacogenomics), may

7.20 Prominent inflammatory infiltrate with eosinophils in the adventitia (**A**) and alveolar attachments of the parenchyma to the outer side (adventitia) of the airway (**B**) in small airways in fatal asthma.

lead to better characterization of the heterogeneous manifest-ations of asthma in individual patients. As most therapies generally used are still symptomatic, these improved insights may allow more personalized therapeutic intervention, at earlier stages of disease, and may even allow development of prevention strategies.

Further reading

Holgate ST, Church MK, Lichtenstein LM (2000). *Allergy*, 2nd edition. CV Mosby, London.

Holgate ST, Holloway J, Wilson S, Bucchieri F, Puddicombe S, Davies DE (2004). Epithelial–mesenchymal communication in the pathogenesis of chronic asthma. *Proc Am Thorac Soc*, 1(2):93–98.

Homer RJ, Elias JA (2005). Airway remodeling in asthma: therapeutic implications of mechanisms. *Physiology*, 20(1): 28–35.

James A (2005). Airway remodeling in asthma. *Curr Opin Pulm Med*, 11(1):1–6.

Jeffery PK (2004). Remodeling and inflammation of bronchi in asthma and chronic obstructive pulmonary disease. *Proc Am Thorac Soc*, 1(3):176–183.

Kumar V, Fausto N, Abbas A (eds) (2004). *Robbins & Cotran's Pathologic Basis of Disease*, 7th edition. WB Saunders Company, New York.

Ten Hacken NHT, Postma DS, Timens W (2003). Airway remodelling and long-term decline in lung function in asthma. *Curr Opin Pulm Med*, 9:9–14.

van Oosterhout AJM, Bloksma N (2005). Regulatory T-lymphocytes in asthma. *Eur Resp J*, 26(5):918–932.

van Rijt LS, Lambrecht BN (2005). Dendritic cells in asthma: a function beyond sensitization. *Clin Exp Allergy*, 35(9):1125–1134.

Ward C, Walters H (2005). Airway wall remodelling: the influence of corticosteroids. *Curr Opin Allergy Clin Immunol*, 5(1):43–48.

Wenzel S. Severe asthma in adults (2005). *Am J Respir Crit Care Med*, 172(2):149–160.

Treatment of Stable Asthma

Dominick Shaw, Pranab Haldar and Ian Pavord

Introduction

Asthma is one of the most prevalent chronic disorders; 8 million people in the UK have been diagnosed with asthma. It predominantly affects younger people. Disease-related morbidity impacts significantly on quality of life and contributes to a large proportion of economic and health-care costs. On average, 1400 people die from asthma each year in the UK alone. Most of these deaths are considered preventable.

Asthma is characterized by symptoms mainly caused by widespread but variable airflow limitation and an increase in airway response to a variety of stimuli. Associated with these abnormalities of airway function is airway inflammation (**8.1**), particularly involving eosinophils and mast cells and orchestrated by T cells predominantly producing T helper (Th)2-type cytokines. Airway inflammation, variable airflow obstruction and airway hyper-responsiveness can occur independently or overlap and vary over time. How they contribute to the symptoms and natural history of the disease and how different treatments affect these features is incompletely understood.

Asthma severity, control and exacerbations

When assessing a patient with asthma it is important to draw a distinction between asthma severity, asthma control and asthma exacerbations. Good asthma control is defined as lack of symptoms, normal lifestyle, near normal lung function and lack of morbidity; asthma severity is quantified by the minimum medication (normally inhaled or oral corticosteroids) required to achieve this. Asthma exacerbations

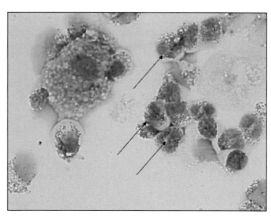

8.1 Eosinophilic inflammation (arrows) in an induced sputum sample from a patient with asthma.

are episodes of increased symptoms and worsening lung function that do not respond adequately to increased use of bronchodilators. Importantly patients with well-controlled or mild asthma may still be vulnerable to (potentially life-threatening) exacerbations.

Overview of asthma management

The goals of asthma treatment are:

- effective control of symptoms, including nocturnal symptoms and exercise-induced asthma
- prevention of exacerbations
- achievement and preservation of best lung function.

These goals should be achieved with minimal side effects from treatment and minimal disruption to the individual's quality of life.

Approach to care

A simplified algorithm summarizing the steps in asthma management is shown in **8.2**. Like all chronic disorders the management of asthma requires a holistic and often multi-disciplinary approach (**8.3**). A patient-centred or a physician-directed approach to care may be appropriate and this will often be governed by disease severity.

Approximately 80% of asthma is managed effectively in primary care. Success is achieved in part through promoting patient education, to increase awareness and understanding of the disease. In most cases of uncomplicated asthma a patient-centred approach is both achievable and desirable, allowing the individual to retain autonomy. The role of the physician in this setting is secondary and may simply

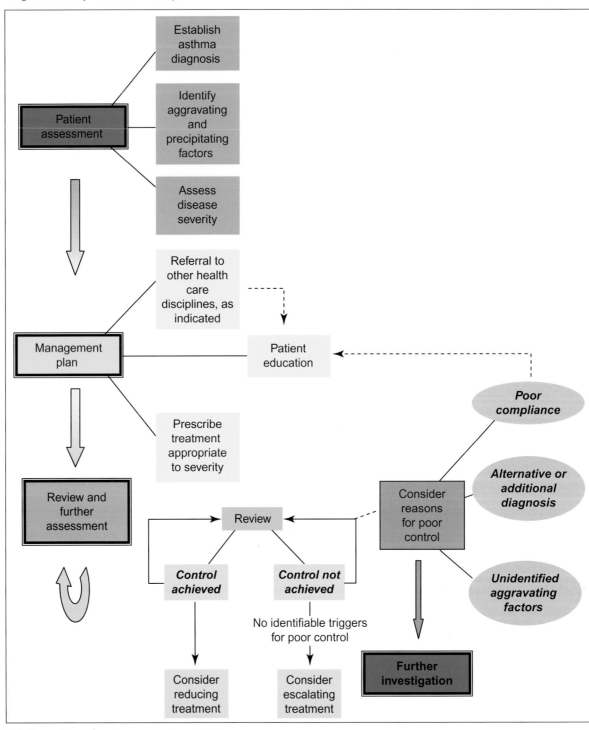

8.2 Overview of asthma management.

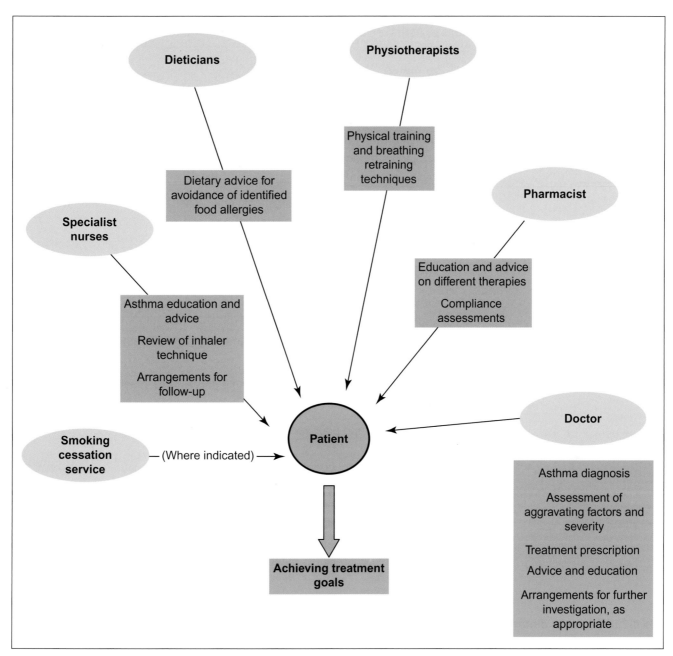

8.3 A multidisciplinary approach to asthma care.

constitute occasional review and availability when concerns or queries arise.

In contrast, the 5–10% of patients with so-called 'refractory' asthma are managed most appropriately by specialists in secondary care. These individuals fail to achieve satisfactory disease control despite maximal or near-maximal pharmacotherapy. They face persistent disease-related morbidity and remain at risk of potentially life-threatening asthma exacerbations. The reason for poor control in these patients is often multifactorial (*Tables 8.1 and 8.2*) and management strategies therefore need to be complex and heterogeneous[1]. The responsible physician must take an active role in identifying aggravating factors and co-morbid conditions that are not readily apparent, in addition to carefully monitoring disease activity and titrating treatment accordingly. Under these circumstances, a physician-led approach to care may be considered more appropriate.

Table 8.1 Common aggravating factors in asthma

Aggravating factor	Comments
Rhinitis	• Avoidance of precipitants such as pollen. • Use of nasal steroids and antihistamine may be helpful.
Gastro oesophageal reflux disease	• Trial of proton pump inhibitor may be considered in patients with suggestive symptoms though trials have not suggested therapeutic efficacy for improving asthma control.
Drugs	• Commonly prescribed medications include aspirin, angiotensin-converting enzyme inhibitors and non-steroidal anti-inflammatory drugs. • All these medications should be withdrawn and replaced with available alternatives if they exacerbate symptoms. • β-Blockers should always be withdrawn.
Common aero-allergens	• Common examples include pollen, pet allergens, house dust mite and fungal spores. • Avoidance measures are recommended though efficacy in improving asthma control is variable.
Smoking	• Smoking cessation should be strongly encouraged and referral to a smoking cessation service is recommended.
Occupational allergens	• Dust, smoke and poor ventilation can all contribute to deterioration in asthma control. • In contrast occupational agents that have been identified in the development of asthma include isocyanates (spray painting); flour; wood dust; glutaraldehyde (nursing); solder/colophony (welding and soldering). • In all cases occupational exposure should be considered and investigated appropriately. Employers have a statutory duty to provide safe employment in cases of occupational asthma.

Table 8.2 Differential diagnosis of asthma

Disorders that may be misdiagnosed as asthma	Disorders likely to co-exist with asthma
Chronic obstructive pulmonary disease.	Dysfunctional breathing disorders, e.g. hyperventilation syndrome.
Bronchiectasis.	Vocal cord dysfunction.
Inhaled foreign body.	Churg–Strauss syndrome
Tumour obstructing proximal airway.	
Left ventricular failure.	

It should be remembered that all the disorders listed as being potentially misdiagnosed as asthma can also co-exist with asthma; these disorders can therefore also contribute to deteriorating control in pre-existing asthma.

Patient education

In all cases patients can play a key role in the management of their asthma and this should be positively encouraged from the outset. Indeed it is well recognized that patients who fail to take an active role in their asthma care make many more emergency care visits and have a higher rate of hospital admissions with recurrent, and often severe, asthma exacerbations. At a minimum, education is necessary to ensure that asthmatic people can fulfil fundamental requirements of their asthma care, notably:

- use of proper inhaler technique (**8.4, 8.5**)
- compliance with prescribed treatment
- avoidance of known asthma triggers or aggravators
- ability to perform peak flow measurements as a guide to disease monitoring (**8.6–8.9**).

Self-management plans

Personal self-management plans contain written instructions and advice that allow individuals to adjust their treatment according to symptoms and peak flow measurements (**8.10**). The instructions given are in accordance with treatment escalation protocols used by physicians and offer an opportunity for patients to retain a degree of autonomy in their disease management. In well-motivated individuals, this strategy has been successful in lowering hospital admission rates for asthma[2].

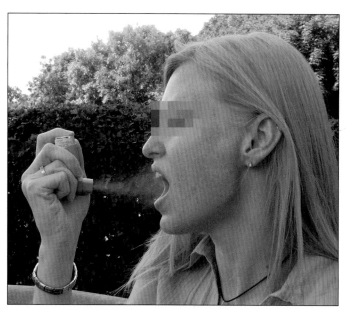

8.5 An example of poor inhaler technique.

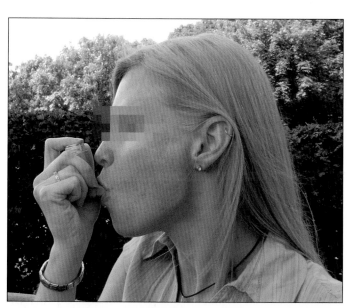

8.4 An example of good inhaler technique, in this case using a salbutamol pressurized metered dose inhaler. Note that inhalation occurs as the inhaler is activated, helping deposition of medication in the lungs.

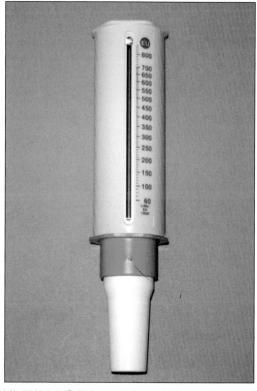

8.6 A Mini-Wright® EU peak flow meter.

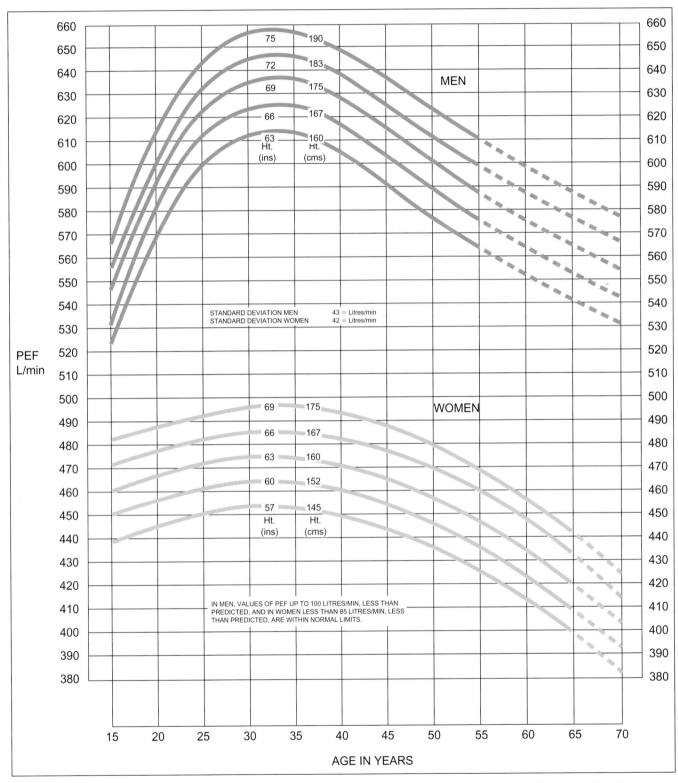

8.7 Predicted peak flow for adults. Reproduced from Nunn AJ, Gregg I (1989). New regression equations for predicting peak expiratory flow in adults. *Br Med J,* **298**:1068–1970.

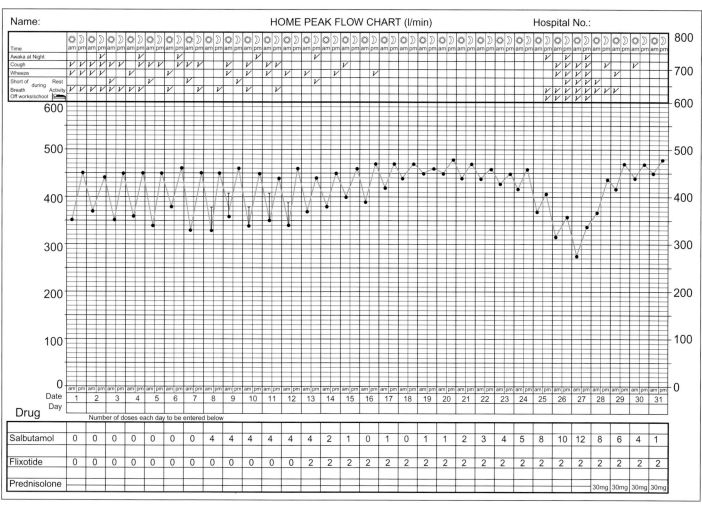

8.8 Peak flow diary of a 30-year-old woman with asthma (height 152 cm). Predicted average peak flow 450 l/min.

Day 1–7: Variable airflow obstruction with a large degree of peak flow variability. Mean peak expiratory flow (PEF) around 400 l/min pre-treatment. High symptom score.

Day 7–12: Salbutamol started. Horizontal lines represent post-bronchodilator (salbutamol) PEF. Note large degree of reversibility to salbutamol, helping confirm diagnosis of asthma. Symptom score improving.

Day 12–19: Inhaled corticosteroid (fluticasone [Flixotide]) started. PEF begins to improve, and diurnal variation decreases. Minimal symptoms, and less bronchodilator use.

Day 19–24: PEF begins to dip. Salbutamol use increases.

Day 24–27: PEF dips to around 60% of predicted for this patient, and symptom scores increase. Oral corticosteroids started. Excess salbutamol use.

Day 27–31: PEF, symptom scores and salbutamol use all improve with oral corticosteroids. Note that inhaled corticosteroids should be continued during an exacerbation, and can be increased two-fold to four-fold.

Non-pharmacological and alternative therapies in asthma

Although pharmacological therapies are central to asthma management, there are several important non-pharmacological measures that do contribute to asthma control. Factors related to patient education including the provision of a self-management plan have already been discussed. However, three interventions merit further consideration:

- smoking cessation
- breathing re-training and Buteyko techniques
- allergen avoidance and immunotherapy.

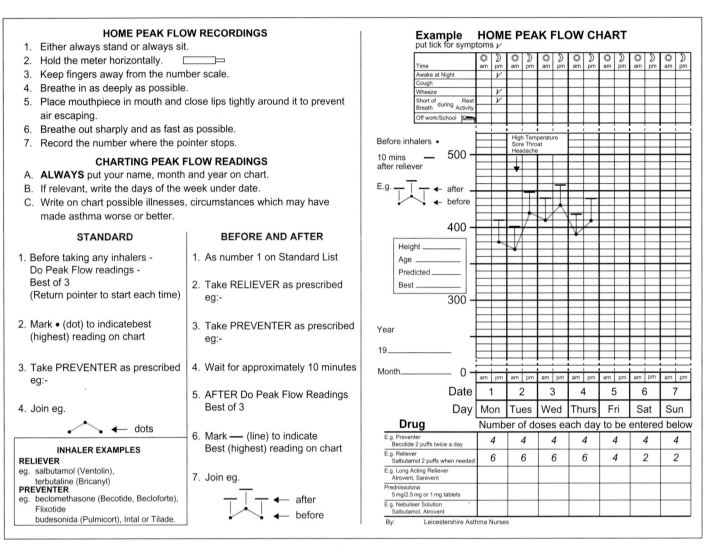

8.9 Back of peak flow diary card, with explanation of peak flow monitoring.

Smoking cessation

Approximately 30% of the UK asthma population are current smokers. The prevalence of smoking is similar to that in the general population. It is well established that patients with asthma who do smoke have an accelerated decline in lung function, increased symptoms and more frequent and severe asthma exacerbations[3]. This was formerly attributed wholly to the irritant effects of tobacco smoke on the airways but it is now also recognized that tobacco smoke reduces the efficacy of asthma treatment, notably inhaled corticosteroids. Patients must therefore be strongly encouraged to stop smoking. Helpful strategies include referral to a smoking cessation clinic that offers both counselling and nicotine replacement therapy as part of a constructive programme.

Breathing re-training and Buteyko techniques

It is well recognized that disordered breathing patterns, of which hyperventilation is an example, can often mimic the clinical features of asthma and should be considered in the differential diagnosis. In addition to being an alternative diagnosis, disordered breathing frequently co-exists in patients with asthma and may contribute significantly to poor symptom control. Physiotherapy based breathing retraining programmes are often effective in resolving this condition. The Buteyko technique is a well-advertised example of such a programme that uses hypoventilation in an effort to raise the partial pressure of carbon dioxide in the blood. This seems to have a beneficial effect on symptoms, and there have been reports of successful reduction in asthma medication requirements[4].

Zone 1

Your asthma is under control if:

- You have no or minimal symptoms during the day or night (wheezing, coughing, short of breath, tightness in chest)
- You can do all of your normal activities without asthma symptoms

Your peak flow reading is [ ] (85% of your best)

Action

Continue to take your usual asthma medicines.

Preventer medicine should be used every day, even when you are feeling well. Your preventer medicine is

name [ ]
colour [ ] Take number of puffs/doses [ ]
dosage [ ] when [ ]

Reliever medicine should be used if you have symptoms, Your reliever medicine is

name [ ]
colour [ ] Take number of puffs/doses [ ]
when [ ]

Other medicines taken regularly may be added tp your treatment if your preventer is not stopping all of your symptoms. Your add-on medicine is name [ ]

colour [ ] Take number of puffs/doses [ ]
when [ ]

If you are always in zone 1, your doctor or nurse may want to reduce (step down) your refular medicines.

Zone 2

Your asthma gets worse if:

- You need to use your reliever inhaler more than once a day
- You have had difficulty sleepin because of your asthma
- Your peak flow reading has fallen to [ ] (between 70% and 85%)

Action

Increase your preventer inhaler

name [ ]
colour [ ] to number of puffs/doses a day [ ]

Stay on this dose until you have had no symptoms for
days [ ] then return to your dose in zone 1.

Continue to take your reliever medicine

name [ ]
colour [ ] when needed.

If your symptoms do not improve in [ ] days contact your doctor or nurse for advice.

Your doctor or nurse will discuss your inhaler with you and check your inhaler technique. You may be started on a different medicine to help to get your symptoms back under control.

If you are often in zone 2, let your doctor or nurse know at your next review. Your usual medicines may need to be increased or changed.

Zone 3

Your asthma is much more severe if:

- You need to take your reliever inhaler every four hours or more often
- You have symptoms all the time
- Your peak flow reading is [ ] and [ ] between (50% and 75%)

Action

Continue taking your preventer medicine as prescribed at the higher dose in zone 2.

Continue taking your reliever medicine when needed.

If you have been prescribed steroid tablets, take
number [ ] 5 mg prednisolone tablets immediately and again every morning for [ ] days or until your symptoms have improved or your peak flow has been at [ ] for two days.

Your doctor or nurse may want you to let them know within 24–36 hours that you have started such a course of tablets. If you regularly take steroid tablets, your doctor will advise you on how to reduce the number you are taking.

If you are often in zone 3, let your doctor or nurse know. Your usual medicines may need to be increased or changed.

Zone 4

It is an asthma emergency if any of the following happen:

1 Your reliever (blue) inhaler does not help
2 Your symptoms get worse (cough, breathless, wheeze, tight chest)
3 You are too breathless to speak
4 Your peak flow reading is below [ ]

Action

1 Take your reliever (blue) inhaler

2 Sit up and loosen tight clothing

3 If no immediate improvement during an attack, continue to take one puff/dose of reliever inhaler every minute for five minutes or until symptoms improve

4 If your symptoms do not improve in five minutes – or if you are in doubt – call 999 or a doctor urgently

Your asthma medicines – what to use on a everyday basis

	Your medicine is:	How much to use:	When to use:	Comments/symptoms:
Preventer				
Reliever				
Other				

How to recognise if your asthma is getting worse

Have you had dufficulty sleeping because of your asthma symptoms (including coughing)?

Have you had your usual asthma symptoms during the day (cough, breathless, wheeze, tight chest)?

Has your asthma interfered with your usual activities (e.g. housework, work or school)?

If 'yes' to one or more of the above, or if you have not seen your doctor or nurse about your asthma for 12 months or more, arrange to have a review, if 'yes' to all of the above – is this an emergency? (see overleaf)

8.10 Asthma Personal Management Plan. Courtesy of Asthma UK.

Allergen avoidance and immunotherapy

Immediate hypersensitivity to airborne allergens is a well-recognized feature among children and young adults with asthma. Allergen exposure can induce bronchospasm, increased bronchial hyper-reactivity and eosinophilic inflammation in susceptible individuals. The term 'extrinsic asthma' was coined to indicate the presumed significance of allergen sensitization in the perpetuation of asthma in these individuals. The profile of allergen sensitization differs geographically according to the prevalence of individual allergens in different areas, although common agents include grass or tree pollen, animal dander or the house dust mite (see **3.1**, **3.5**, **4.9(A)**). Cockroach allergen is particularly common in less affluent regions of North America. Both epidemiological studies and direct bronchial challenge with sensitized allergen suggest a strong causal association between allergen exposure and asthma. Despite this, rather surprisingly, the evidence for improvement in asthma control with allergen avoidance is weak. General measures such as removing animals from direct contact, cleaning to reduce house dust mite numbers and closing windows to reduce pollen exposure are nevertheless recommended by most physicians. Given the lack of efficacy in studies to date, more expensive and disruptive interventions such as the use of special bed covers, chemical or heat cleaning of soft furnishings, air filtering and carpet removal is debatable[5].

Allergen-specific immunotherapy, or desensitization, involves the administration of specific allergen extracts at increasing concentrations over time to induce a state of immunological tolerance. It is a method that is not generally recommended for asthma in the UK and is reserved for those who have a documented severe sensitization to an allergen that is frequently unavoidable and which appears to be having a significant impact on asthma control. It has been used in some patients with severe grass pollen sensitization resulting in a notable improvement of symptoms of allergic rhinitis. Some patients with allergic asthma have also shown an improvement in symptom control and airway responsiveness. However the technique is labour intensive and major concerns about safety remain as life-threatening anaphylactic reactions can occur.

Pharmacological treatment of asthma

The mainstay of asthma treatment is pharmacological therapy, with the introduction of medications in a stepwise fashion in order to maintain asthma control[6]. Classically, asthma medications may be broadly divided into bronchodilator medications such as β-agonists, which relax airway smooth muscle and relieve symptoms, and the anti-inflammatory medications (usually inhaled corticosteroids) that damp down inflammation helping to maintain lung function and prevent exacerbations. Certain drug classes have a dual effect. The relation between symptoms and the severity of the underlying airway inflammation is inconsistent and often unreliable. Most patients with asthma therefore need continual treatment with an anti-inflammatory medication to prevent future exacerbations and decline in lung function, even if they have minimal symptoms.

A bronchodilator should be used to relieve symptoms in any patient who has symptomatic asthma. An anti-inflammatory medication should be considered if a patient has had an exacerbation of asthma in the past 2 years, is using a reliever three times a week or more, is symptomatic three times a week or more, or is waking at least one night a week. If a patient still has poor control after their compliance and exact diagnosis has been checked, further medication can be added, or the dose of inhaled corticosteroid increased.

Bronchodilators

Short acting β-agonists (SABAs)

SABAs such as salbutamol or terbutaline lead to bronchodilatation and improvement in lung function. They provide rapid relief of symptoms by relaxing airway smooth muscle. Short-acting inhaled β-agonists are also used for the treatment of acute exacerbations of asthma and are useful for the pre-treatment of exercise-induced asthma. They are generally very safe but side effects can include tachycardia and muscle tremor.

Long acting β-agonists (LABAs)

LABAs such as salmeterol and formoterol have a comparable mechanism of action and side effect profile to SABAs. These inhaled medications are usually started if a patient has poor control despite using a SABA and inhaled corticosteroid.

Salmeterol has a slower onset of action than formoterol, but both medications are available in combination form with an inhaled corticosteroid, improving patient compliance with steroid therapy.

Methylxanthines

Methylxanthines (like theophylline) are pharmacological agents that work by phosphodiesterase inhibition. This pathway is associated primarily with bronchodilatation by relaxation of airway smooth muscle. However, studies also indicate that they have weak anti-inflammatory effects. Theophyllines are used via the oral route in stable asthma, but can also be used intravenously in the treatment of acute asthma. Levels should be monitored as systemic side effects can occur with higher plasma levels. The side effects are usually preceded by nausea and vomiting. Specific inhibitors of phosphodiesterase type 4 such as roflumilast and cilomilast may be more effective but their role in the management of asthma remains to be defined.

Anti-inflammatories

Inhaled corticosteroids

Inhaled corticosteroids such as fluticasone, budesonide, beclomethasone, mometasone and ciclesonide all work by damping down inflammation in the airways of the lung. They are the most effective treatment in persistent asthma and are the backbone of all treatment protocols. There is still debate about when exactly to start inhaled corticosteroids[7], but in general they should be used if patients who are not controlled on a short acting β₂-agonist are using inhaled β₂-agonists three times a week or more, or are symptomatic three times a week or more, or waking one night a week. As they are inhaled their side effects are mostly limited to local problems with oral *Candida* infection and dysphonia being the commonest. However some systemic effects such as skin bruising, cataracts and osteopenia may occur, particularly if used in doses over 1600 μg/day (beclomethasone dipropionate equivalents), so they should be used at the lowest possible dose while maintaining asthma control.

Leukotriene modifiers

Leukotriene modifiers are a class of anti-asthmatic drugs that include cysteinyl leukotriene 1 receptor antagonists (montelukast, pranlukast, zafirlukast) and the 5-lipoxygenase inhibitor (zileuton). These drugs have mild anti-inflammatory effects and also cause some bronchodilatation. There are relatively few class-specific side effects. The exact place of the leukotriene modifiers in asthma management protocols is unclear; they may be of particular benefit in asthma associated with rhinitis or in aspirin-induced asthma where there is evidence of cysteinyl leukotriene overproduction. In view of the relative paucity of side effects associated with this class of drugs, they are frequently tried in younger children to aid disease control and as a steroid-sparing agent.

Oral corticosteroids

Oral corticosteroids (typically prednisolone) are usually reserved for the treatment of acute asthma exacerbations. They are also used in patients whose asthma is not controlled despite full treatment with other asthma medications. Oral corticosteroids work in a manner similar to inhaled corticosteroids, but they have systemic effects, as well as anti-inflammatory effects in the lung. There is evidence emerging that when compared with inhaled corticosteroids, oral corticosteroids reach the more distal lung perhaps explaining their beneficial effect in more severe asthma[8]. Oral corticosteroids can cause osteoporosis, hypertension, diabetes, hypothalamic–pituitary–adrenal axis suppression, cataracts, glaucoma, obesity, skin thinning and muscle weakness.

Patients with asthma who are on long-term systemic glucocorticosteroids should receive prophylactic treatment against osteoporosis.

Anti IgE

Omalizumab, an antibody against IgE, has shown benefit in a subset of patients with severe allergic asthma and has now received a licence for use in this cohort.

Asthma treatment protocols (8.11)

Various treatment protocols exist. All are based on the stepwise increase or decrease of asthma medication; stepping up or down is dependent on two factors:

- presence of asthma control
- frequency of asthma exacerbations.

Asthma control can be easily and reliably gauged by asking three simple questions:

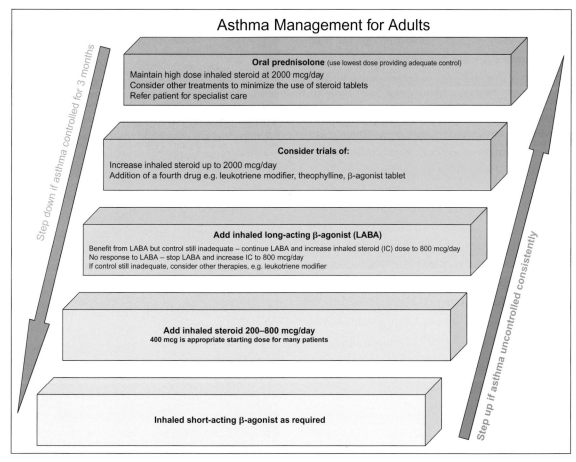

8.11 Asthma treatment protocol for adults.

- Are you waking at night due to your asthma?
- How often are you using your reliever (salbutamol/ terbutaline) a day?
- Is your asthma interfering with your work/normal daily activities?

If the answer to any of these questions is yes, then treatment needs to be increased. If the patient answers no to all these questions over a period of at least 3 months, then treatment may be stepped down. Occasionally, apparently usually well-controlled patients can have frequent asthma exacerbations. These patients should also have their treatment increased.

Peak flow monitoring

Asthma exacerbations may be predicted by monitoring a patient's peak expiratory flow (PEF) using a peak flow meter (**8.6–8.9**). PEF represents the highest airflow velocity transiently achieved during a forced expiration. Flow is inversely related to airway resistance. The majority of resistance occurs in the proximal airways and the PEF therefore corresponds well to large airway patency. Patients should record the best of three peak flow measurements performed in quick succession at least once a day, though measurements undertaken in the morning and evening will provide information on diurnal variability. The value obtained for PEF should then be compared to the predicted or best ever value for the patient. The best ever value is often considered more representative to the individual but in some circumstances PEF measurements have never been recorded during periods of good asthma control. Under these circumstances, the predicted value is preferable. If measured PEF is less than 75% of the target PEF for the patient, the inhaled corticosteroid dose should be doubled or quadrupled. If the value falls to less than 60%, oral steroids should be considered whereas values less than 50% indicate an acute severe exacerbation that may warrant hospital admission. PEF monitoring is especially useful in patients who have poor perception of their symptoms.

Modes of delivery

Different inhalers deliver different drugs in various ways, and understanding and remembering all the types of inhaler is not always easy. The two most important factors when choosing an inhaler are ensuring good inhaler technique and checking for poor compliance. Both of these factors are closely related to patient preference.

The most common form of inhaler is the pressurized metered dose inhaler (pMDI). These inhalers are commonly used with spacer devices. Spacers help prevent oropharyngeal medication deposition and problems with inhalation co-ordination. (**8.12, 8.13**). Breath-activated inhalers and dry powdered inhalers are also designed to help prevent these two common problems (**8.14–8.20**). Every time an inhaler is issued the patient's inhaler technique should be checked. If it is found to be poor a different medication delivery device should be used. Compliance can be checked in several ways: checking with the dispensing pharmacist

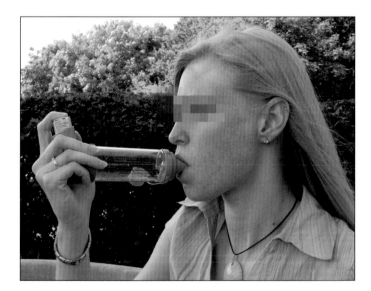

8.12 A salbutamol pressurized metered dose inhaler used with a spacer. This helps prevent oropharyngeal deposition of medication and obviates the need for good co-ordination.

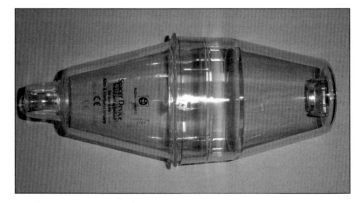

8.13 Another type of spacer device.

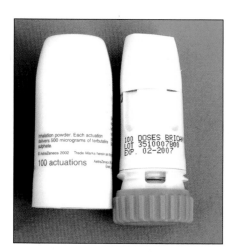

8.14 Terbutaline is a bronchodilator. The Turbohaler® needs less co-ordination and dexterity to use than a pressurized metered dose inhaler.

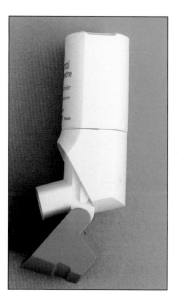

8.15 A salbutamol breath-activated inhaler. Less dexterity and co-ordination is needed to use this inhaler.

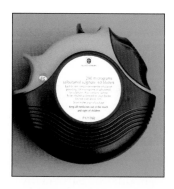

8.16 Salbutamol is a bronchodilator used for symptom relief. The Accuhaler® requires less co-ordination and dexterity to use.

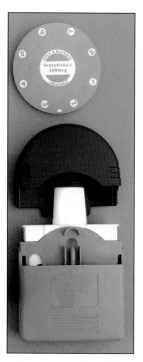

8.17 A salbutamol Diskhaler® needs manual dexterity to use, but less inhalation co-ordination.

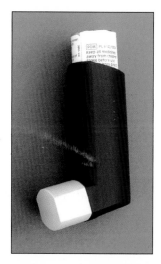

8.18 Beclomethasone dipropionate: an inhaled corticosteroid with a dose of 100 μg/activation. The inhaler is a pressurized metered dose inhaler. Compare inhaler colour to that in **8.19**.

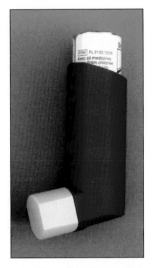

8.19 Beclomethasone dipropionate: an inhaled corticosteroid with a dose of 250 μg/activation. The inhaler is a pressurized metered dose inhaler.

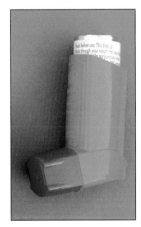

8.20 Fluticasone pressurized metered dose inhaler. Fluticasone is a more potent form of inhaled corticosteroid, and in general only half as much should be prescribed compared with beclomethasone or budesonide.

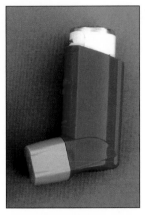

8.21 Seretide (fluticasone/salmeterol) combines both the inhaled corticosteroid fluticasone and the long-acting β-agonist salmeterol in the same inhaler.

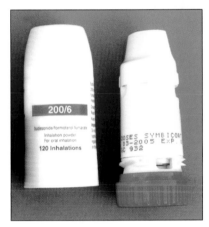

8.22 A Turbohaler®, combining budesonide (an inhaled corticosteroid) and formoterol (a long-acting β-agonist).

that the medications prescribed are being collected is by far the simplest method. Other methods used include weighing the canisters and checking blood theophylline and prednisolone levels, if appropriate.

Combination inhalers

Recently, combination inhalers have been used more frequently in the treatment of asthma (**8.21**, **8.22**). These inhalers consist of an inhaled corticosteroid combined with a long-acting β-agonist. Combination inhalers have consistently been shown to reduce asthma exacerbations and they may also improve treatment compliance. The Symbicort® Turbohaler can be used for both immediate relief and prevention of symptoms. This approach, called single inhaler therapy, may be particularly useful for patients with poor compliance and has been associated with a significant reduction in asthma exacerbations in a randomized controlled study[9].

Special situations

Pregnancy

During pregnancy about one-third of asthma patients experience an improvement in their asthma, one-third experience a worsening of symptoms and one-third remain the same. Interestingly mothers carrying female babies appear to have more symptoms and need more steroid courses than those carrying male babies. This may reflect the higher levels of intrinsic immunosuppression associated with carrying the male fetus. Uncontrolled asthma during pregnancy presents a risk to both mother and baby; fortunately most asthma medications are safe during pregnancy. Importantly, the risk of harm to the fetus from severe or chronically under-treated asthma outweighs any small risk from the medications used to control asthma. The only medications that should not be started during pregnancy are the leukotriene modifiers, as these have limited safety data in pregnancy.

Exercise-induced asthma

The prevalence of exercise-induced asthma varies from 7% to more than 20% in the general population. Most patients are controlled with as required use of short-acting β-agonists during exercise; the leukotriene modifiers, long-acting β-agonists and the prophylactic use of inhaled sodium cromoglycate can be tried if control is not achieved. Antihistamines and anticholinergics are of no benefit.

Hypertension

The treatment of hypertension and heart disease can present a problem in asthma as β-blockers can cause bronchoconstriction and exacerbate asthma. Calcium-channel blockers (such as amlodipine) have the theoretical advantages of opposing contraction in tracheobronchial smooth muscle and inhibiting mast cell degranulation. Consequently the use of a calcium-channel blocker alone or with a low dose of thiazide diuretic represents the preferred regimen for the initial management of hypertension and asthma. Occasionally angiotensin-converting enzyme inhibitors can exacerbate cough variant asthma and in this situation they should be swapped to angiotensin receptor II antagonists.

Future strategies in asthma management

Although corticosteroids are effective anti-inflammatory agents that have revolutionized treatment protocols for asthma since the 1960s, concerns over their long-term use remain and include the following:

- Patients at the severe end of the asthma spectrum require maintenance oral corticosteroid therapy that is commonly associated with significant side effects.
- Despite the use of oral corticosteroids, some patients do not achieve satisfactory asthma control and remain at risk of life-threatening exacerbations.
- Although considered relatively safe, the effect of chronic inhaled corticosteroid therapy, particularly at higher doses in children, may be associated with side effects seen with oral therapy.

Two different strategies are presently under development that may help address these concerns:

- targeted steroid therapy that is titrated to the level of underlying airway inflammation
- monoclonal antibody therapies that specifically inhibit inflammatory pathways implicated in asthma.

Monitoring of airway inflammation

Monitoring disease activity in patients with asthma that is difficult to control is of primary importance. A conventional approach to disease monitoring (i.e. symptoms and peak flows) may be inadequate either because patients do not comply with performing and documenting peak flow measurements or because levels of underlying airway inflammation do not correlate with symptoms. Despite having good day-to-day control of symptoms, a subgroup of brittle asthmatics are characterized by sudden and severe asthma exacerbations. The majority of these patients are found to have high levels of active eosinophilic inflammation that seems to correlate closely with susceptibility to asthma exacerbations.

An alternative way to monitor disease activity is therefore to monitor levels of eosinophilic airway inflammation and prescribe steroid therapy according to the level of airway eosinophilia. Over the past decade, a method known as *sputum induction* has been developed that enables non-invasive sampling of lower airway secretions. The technique involves expectoration of sputum by patients following nebulization of hypertonic saline and samples are then processed and examined under a microscope. Eosinophilic inflammation (**8.1**) may be expressed as a percentage of the total cell count.

A randomized controlled trial that compared titrated steroid therapy (to maintain sputum eosinophil counts below 3%) with a conventional protocol (British Thoracic Society guidelines) has demonstrated a significantly lower exacerbation frequency, without requiring a higher total steroid dose, over 12 months in the group managed by monitoring airway inflammation[10]. These results indicate the value of having a direct and objective measure of airway inflammation. As sputum induction is a fairly specialized and labour-intensive technique, surrogate markers of eosinophilic airway inflammation are being sought. Of these, the most promising to date has been the measurement of fractional exhaled nitric oxide (FeNO). Studies have demonstrated a significant correlation between FeNO levels and underlying airway eosinophilia, measured by sputum induction and bronchoscopically. However, clinical trials utilizing FeNO to titrate inhaled corticosteroid dosing have succeeded only in maintaining asthma control at lower doses of maintenance inhaled corticosteroids without significantly impacting on the frequency of asthma exacerbations.[11] Furthermore, a proportion of the asthma population display high levels of FeNO without significant eosinophilic airway inflammation. The place of FeNO in the management of asthma therefore remains unclear. It is however likely that the future will see monitoring of airway inflammation being incorporated within asthma management protocols.

Monoclonal antibody therapy

Based on the presumed underlying immunopathogenesis, monoclonal antibody therapies have now been developed against the key pro-inflammatory mediators thought to be responsible for perpetuating airway inflammation in asthma. The use of etanercept, a monoclonal antibody to the tumour necrosis factor α receptor, has shown promising results in the control of refractory asthma symptoms by improving airway hyper-responsiveness[12]. Trials with antibodies to interleukin-5 and interleukin-4 are also underway. All these engineered molecular therapies are very selective in their mode of action and the cost of therapy is very high. For both of these reasons it is likely that their use will be limited to a carefully selected population who are most likely to benefit.

Conclusion

The management of stable asthma is based on scientific principles that govern the stepwise methodical use of available treatment options. Although such an approach is effective in the large majority of asthmatic people, a minority of patients with severe disease continue to account for a large proportion of asthma-related morbidity and mortality. Research at both a clinical and molecular level is seeking to identify novel therapeutic options and alternative strategies that may address this ongoing deficiency.

References

1. Heaney LG, Robinson DS (2005). Severe asthma treatment: need for characterising patients. *Lancet*, **365**(9463):974–976.
2. Toelle BG, Ram FS (2004). Written individualised management plans for asthma in children and adults. *Cochrane Database Syst Rev*, 2:CD002171.
3. Thomson NC, Chaudhuri R, Livingston E (2004). Asthma and cigarette smoking. *Eur Respir J*, **24**(5):822–833.
4. Bowler SD, Green A, Mitchell C (1998). Buteyko breathing techniques in asthma: a blinded randomised controlled trial. *Med J Aust*, **169**:575–578.
5. Woodcock A, Forster L, Matthews E, Martin J, Letley L, Vickers M, Britton J, Strachan D, Howarth P, Altmann D, Frost C, Custovic A; Medical Research Council General Practice Research Framework (2003). Control of exposure to mite allergen and allergen-impermeable bed covers for adults with asthma. *N Engl J Med*, **349**(3):225–236.
6. British Guideline on the Management of Asthma (2003). *Thorax*, **58**:(Suppl I).
7. Boushey HA (2005). Daily inhaled corticosteroid should not be prescribed for mild persistent asthma. A pro con debate. *Am J Respir Crit Care Med*, **172**(4):412–414.
8. Barnes PJ (2004). Corticosteroid resistance in airways disease. *Proc Am Thorac Soc* **1**(3):264–268.
9. O'Byrne PM, Bisgaard H, Godard PP, Pistolesi M, Palmqvist M, Zhu Y, Ekstrom T, Bateman ED (2005). Budesonide/Formoterol combination therapy as both maintenance and reliever medication in asthma. *Am J Respir Crit Care Med*, **171**(2):129–136.
10. Green RH, Brightling CE, McKenna S, Hargadon B, Parker D, Bradding P, Wardlaw AJ, Pavord ID (2002). Asthma exacerbations and sputum eosinophil counts: a randomised controlled trial. *Lancet*, **360**(9347):1715–1721.

11. Smith AD, Cowan JO, Brassett KP, Herbison GP, Taylor DR (2005). Use of exhaled nitric oxide measurements to guide treatment in chronic asthma. *N Engl J Med*, **352**(21):2163–2173.

12. Berry MA, Hargadon B, Shelley M, Parker D, Shaw DE, Green RH, Bradding P, Brightling CE, Wardlaw AJ, Pavord ID (2006). Evidence for a role of tumour necrosis factor alpha in refractory asthma. *N Engl J Med*, **354**(7):697–708.

Further reading

British Guideline on the Management of Asthma: a national clinical guideline. British Thoracic Society and Scottish Intercollegiate Guidelines Network. Revised edition, April 2004 (www.brit-thoracic.org).

Global Strategy for Asthma Management and Prevention. Updated 2003. NIH publication NO 02–3659 (www.ginasthma.com).

Useful Contacts

British Thoracic Society (www.brit-thoracic.org.uk)
American Thoracic Society (www.thoracic.org)
Asthma UK (www.asthma.org.uk)

Chapter 9

Assessment and Management of Patients with Acute Asthma

Al Ajmi Mubarak, N Behbehani and J M FitzGerald

Background

In recent years there has been an increased prevalence of asthma. It is estimated that around 300 million people in the world currently have asthma and it is expected that this will have increased to 400 million by 2025. In the USA, asthma represents the eleventh most frequent diagnosis (illness or injury) in the emergency department. Furthermore the economic cost of asthma is substantial, amounting to US$12.7 billion in the USA.

Asthma is a disease characterized by chronic airways inflammation and variable airways obstruction leading to persistent symptoms as well as intermittent acute exacerbations especially in the absence of regular anti-inflammatory treatment (**9.1, 9.2**). In a recent prospective study of over 1000 patients in multiple locations we have shown significant care gaps persist across a wide range of health delivery systems from high- to low-income countries. Healthcare costs associated with acute asthma are also significant and often underestimate the impact especially from a societal perspective.

Self-medication not only depends on the severity of the exacerbation but also on the healthcare setting, availability and access to primary and secondary healthcare. Patients with increasing asthma symptoms may self-medicate, visit their primary care physician or present to their nearest hospital for emergency care. Hence we believe that assessment and management of acute exacerbation should ideally start from the home. This can be achieved in the form of a written action plan (**9.3**), reinforced by patient education, anti-inflammatory medication and regular follow-up. Appropriate assessment, regular bronchodilator therapy, controlled oxygen and systemic corticosteroids are the principles of management of acute asthma.

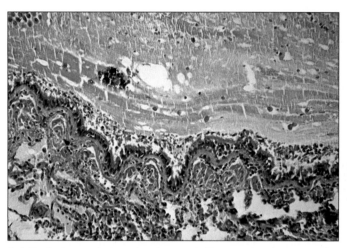

9.1 Pathology of chronic airways inflammation in asthma.

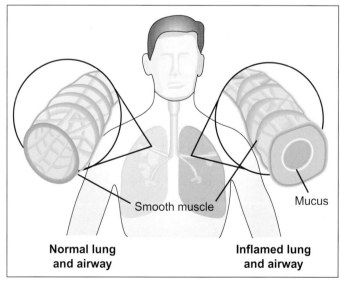

9.2 Inflamed airway versus normal airway.

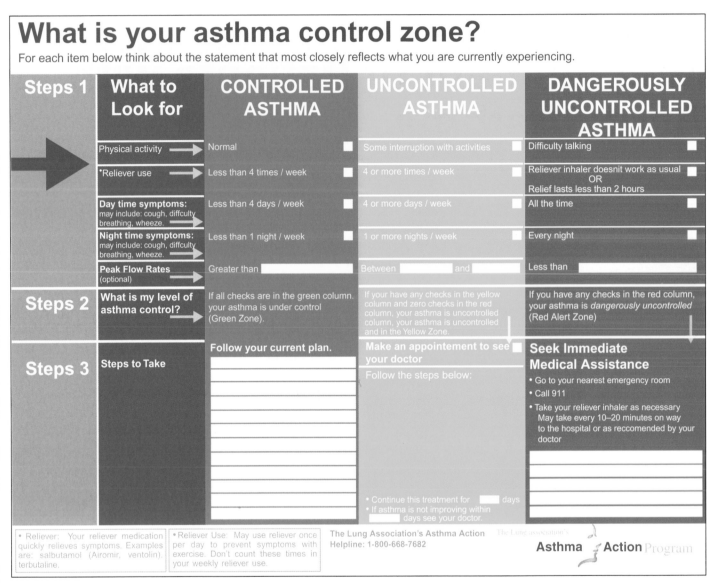

9.3 A typical action plan showing how patients should respond to a worsening of their asthma.

Classification of acute asthma

A classification of the severity of acute asthma has been developed and agreed on based on consensus. This classification system uses a combination of physical findings (speech, breathlessness in relation to position, level of consciousness, respiratory rate, heart rate, accessory muscle use, severity of wheezing) and peak expiratory flow rate (PEFR) after initial treatment (*Table 9.1*).

Assessment of acute exacerbation of asthma

To assess an acute exacerbation of asthma, initial (static) assessment and an assessment after treatment (dynamic) are required. The assessment should include a clinical component (history and physical examination); measurement of airflow obstruction and the measurement of oxygen saturation and in more severe attacks the assessment of alveolar ventilation with arterial blood gas measurements.

Table 9.1 Stratification of the severity of an asthma attack based upon symptoms and physical examination

Imminent	Severe	Moderate	Mild	Sign
	On lying down	On talking Prefers to sit up	On walking Can lie down	Breathlessness
Cannot speak	Words	Parts of phrases	Phrases	Speaking
Sleepy or confused	Always agitated Often >30/min	Usually agitated Increased	May be agitated Increased	Level of consciousness Breathing rate
Paradoxical	Usually	Usually	No	Muscle retraction
Absent	Very strong	Strong	Moderate	Wheezing
Bradycardia	>120	100–120	<100	Pulse/min
Impossible to measure	<50%; <100 l/min	50–70%	Over 70%	Peak expiratory flow after treatment

Medical history

A brief pertinent history is needed to evaluate the patient, looking for a history of prior mechanical ventilation for asthma, excessive use of β-agonists, a very rapid onset, psychosocial problems and a history of non-adherence, which all have been identified as markers for severe asthma and risk factors for near-fatal and fatal asthma.

Physical examination

Signs that indicate severe asthma include:

- inability to lie supine and diaphoresis which correlate well with PEFR measurement
- respiratory rate >30/min
- heart rate >120/min
- pulsus paradoxus (PP) >12 mmHg.

However, these parameters are quite variable in acute asthma and absence of these levels should not be taken as evidence against the presence of a severe attack. PP is an accentuation of the normal inspiratory reduction in stroke volume due to large negative intra-pleural pressure generated during vigorous aspiratory effort in acute severe asthma. Despite PP having been shown to be a valuable sign indicating asthma severity, it is not easy or accurate to measure using a sphygmomanometer. PP also falls in fatiguing patients unable to generate strong inspiratory effort, which may be wrongly

taken as a sign of improvement. Physical examination should include examination for stridor, which may indicate upper airway obstruction (this may mimic asthma), asymmetrical breath sounds and subcutaneous emphysema that may indicate the presence of pneumothorax or barotrauma. Cyanosis is a very imperfect clinic sign but its absence should not be interpreted as a sign of mild to moderate exacerbation.

Airflow obstruction measurement

Wheezing is the clinical sign resulting from airway obstruction in asthma (although it can also be found in chronic obstructive lung disease). Shim and colleagues showed that expiratory wheeze is associated with a higher PEFR than biphasic wheeze (inspiratory and expiratory). However the overall correlation of wheeze with the degree of airway obstruction is poor and patients with severe obstruction may have a silent chest. This emphasizes the need for objective measurement of airway obstruction using either PEFR or forced expiratory volume in one second (FEV_1). Both methods are effort dependent and need good co-operation and technique. PEFR is easier to measure and requires small, relatively cheap equipment (**9.4**). There is good correlation between PEFR and FEV_1 in acute and non-acute asthma (**9.5**). Ideally, PEFR or FEV_1 should be measured before and after treatment but without causing a significant delay in the initiation of treatment. There is a very small risk that the measurement of PEFR or FEV_1 in patients with severe obstruction may lead to a worsening in airflow obstruction. However, this manoeuvre is safe in most patients with acute asthma (**9.6–9.8**). It is clearly useful to measure PEFR after treatment. Stein and colleagues showed that PEFR at presentation did not predict the patients who needed admission. However, PEFR 2 hours after treatment was more useful in predicting the need for admission. Similar results were obtained by other groups, which showed that PEFR at 30 minutes and FEV_1 at 1 hour were better predictors of the need for hospital admission than initial measurements.

Arterial blood gas analysis and oximetry

With the availability of objective measures of airway obstruction the need for arterial blood gas analysis in acute asthma has diminished significantly. Nowak and colleagues have shown that $FEV_1 >25\%$ predicted rules out hypercapnoea or significant hypoxaemia, and similar findings were obtained using PEFR measurement. Mountain and colleagues have shown that the pattern of abnormal arterial blood gases in adult patients presenting with acute asthma to the emergency department was: simple respiratory alkalosis 48%, respiratory acidosis 26% and metabolic acidosis either simple or as part of mixed disturbance with respiratory acidosis 28%. The mechanism of metabolic acidosis in acute asthma is not clear but it is postulated to be secondary to lactate accumulation.

Pulse oximetry is a very simple and quick way to assess oxygen saturation in bronchial asthma. Initial measurement at room air should be done before starting oxygen therapy. It

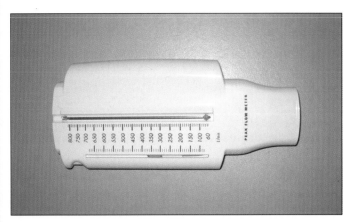

9.4 A peak flow meter which may be used by the patient or a healthcare worker to assess the severity of an acute asthma attack.

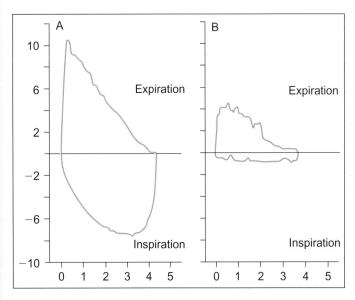

9.5 Two examples of spirometry (A) showing a normal flow-volume loop and (B) showing severe airflow obstruction.

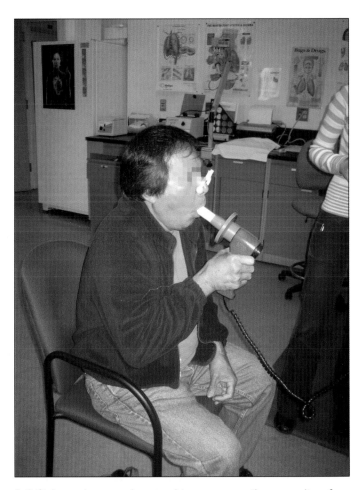

9.6 Spirometry may be used to measure the severity of airflow obstruction.

helps to determine the need for oxygen supplementation and alleviates the need for more invasive arterial blood gas analysis in a large percentage of patients. Carruthers and colleagues have shown that when oxygen saturation on room air was higher than 92% at presentation, the likelihood of respiratory failure defined by blood gas analysis is <5%. Furthermore, oxygen saturation has been shown to predict poor outcome or the need for more intensive treatment in children.

Chest radiography

Several studies showed that unselected routine chest X-rays in acute asthma have a very low yield. Zieverink and colleagues found abnormalities in only 2.2% of 528 chest X-rays taken in a group of 122 asthma patients presenting to the emergency department. Hence, chest X-rays should be reserved for patients who fail to respond to initial treatment especially in the presence of signs suggestive of barotraumas, localizing signs suggestive of either pneumonia or collapse, or when diagnosis other than asthma, e.g. pulmonary oedema, is suspected.

Patient outcome prediction

In a study by Rodrigo and colleagues using factor analysis the authors identified a four-factor solution for the assessment of acute asthma. The first factor is related to measurement of airway obstruction (PEFR, FEV_1, forced vital capacity (FVC) and percent variation of FEV_1 at 30 minutes over baseline), the second factor included respiratory rate, accessory muscle use and level of dyspnoea, the third factor included heart rate and wheezing, and the fourth factor contained demographic variables including age, duration of attack and steroid use. The result of this factor analysis indicated that acute asthma is a multidimensional problem and these objective and subjective variables represent separate and non-overlapping dimensions.

A two-item bedside acute asthma index based on PEFR as percentage of predicted value and PEFR variation of baseline both measured at 30 minutes after initial treatment has been shown to be useful in prediction of poor response early in acute asthma. The acute asthma score ranged from 0 to 4 and a score of 4 (which means PEFR at 30 minutes <40% predicted) and a change from baseline <60 l/min had a positive predicted value of 0.84 in predicting a poor response to emergency department treatment and hence the need for admission.

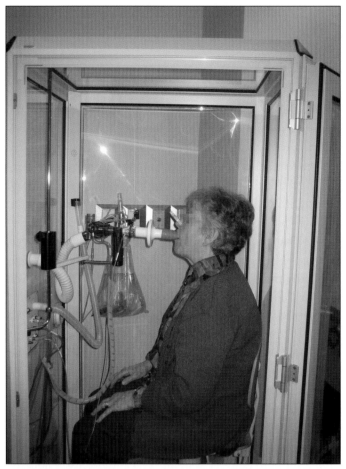

9.7 Detailed lung function carried out in a body box may be useful in some asthma patients to rule out other pulmonary conditions.

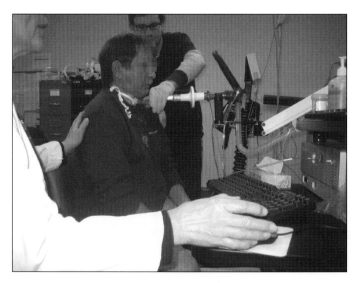

9.8 Spirometry in a patient with tracheostomy.

Another attempt at predicting poor outcome was made and an index was derived based on PEFR as percentage of predicted and use of accessory muscle at 60 minutes. The index ranged from 0 to 2 (a score of 2 means the presence of both factors: a PEFR at 60 minutes ≤40% predicted and accessory muscle use, whereas a score of 0 means absence of both at 60 minutes). A score of 0 or 2 were good in predicting good and poor response to emergency department treatment, respectively. However a score of 1(which means either variable present) was poor in predicting the outcome. Most of the patients in this study had a score of 1 hence it was difficult to predict outcome based on a severity score measured at 60 minutes for the majority of patients.

In summary, it is difficult to find a single predictor for the need of hospital admission. We feel that patients with PEFR >60% predicted or personal best after 1–2 hours of treatment can be safely discharged from the emergency department with appropriate anti-inflammatory medicines and follow-up and patients with PEFR <40% should be admitted to hospital for more intensive treatment. The patients who have PEFR between 40% and 60% need to be evaluated for other risk factors of severity and identified risks of mortality from asthma (**9.9**). These patients will probably need a longer duration of treatment in the emergency department with serial measurement of PEFR or spirometry to better determine their outcome.

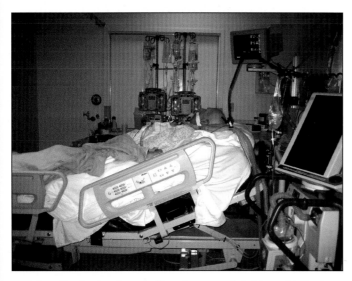

9.9 A patient who has suffered a near-fatal heart attack receiving mechanical ventilation.

Treatment of acute asthma

Bronchodilators

Initial treatment of asthma should be started concurrently during the assessment of patients with acute asthma as outlined above. Regular short-acting β-agonists should be given in all cases; ipratropium bromide can be added in moderate to severe attacks only. There appears to be no additional benefit derived from continuous versus intermittent delivery of bronchodilator treatment. One systematic review found no significant difference in admission rate between 1 hour of continuous nebulization and 2 hours of intermittent nebulized salbutamol (relative risk [RR] 0.68; 95% confidence interval [CI] 0.33 to 1.38). The recommended dose is usually in the range of 2.5–5 mg of salbutamol diluted in 2.5 ml of saline. The randomized controlled trials (RCTs) included in the review also used systemic steroids. Subsequent RCTs similarly found no significant difference in lung function or rate of hospital admission in subjects treated with either continuous or intermittent salbutamol.

Several studies including two systematic reviews have shown the delivery of bronchodilator with either a spacing device (**9.10, 9.11**) or a nebulizer to be equivalent (**9.12**). In one systematic review of 13 RCTs the outcome was similar for both delivery systems. The authors also evaluated patients with more severe airflow obstruction and found no difference in outcomes. In this sub-analysis, patients with an FEV_1 less than 30% predicted were excluded. Because of the differences in symptom scores, which were measured on different scales, the findings could not be combined, and comparisons based on symptoms could not be done. There were no differences in safety parameters between both groups. One systematic review showed no benefit of the routine use of intravenous bronchodilator therapy compared with the use of the inhaled route (see **8.14–22** for examples of different types of inhalers).

Ipratropium bromide

The role of ipratropium bromide in acute asthma was evaluated in two systemic reviews. A marginal additional bronchodilator effect was shown in individual studies; the systematic reviews have been helpful in identifying a subset of patients in whom the combination of treatments was associated with a reduction in hospitalization as well as an additional bronchodilator effect in the presence of severe airflow obstruction. The impact was clinically significant with an odds ratio

(OR) of 0.62 (95% CI 0.44 to 0.88). Evaluating patients with more severe airflow obstruction defined as an FEV_1 less than 30% predicted found that additional treatment with ipratropium significantly improved FEV_1 over 90 minutes. The second systematic review confirmed these results. The most recently published systematic review further supports the use of ipratropium bromide in moderate to severe acute asthma attacks. A more recent RCT compared salbutamol alone with salbutamol combined with ipratropium. It found that adding ipratropium significantly improved the PEFR (and it also showed a reduction in the proportion of patients admitted to hospital (20% with ipratropium *vs* 39% with placebo, $P < 0.01$). Traditionally, nebulized therapy has been

administered in saline delivery systems but the most recently published systematic review to address this issue has shown that the use of magnesium sulphate as a delivery vehicle is associated with better lung function and a trend towards a reduction in hospitalizations. The usual recommended dose is 0.25 mg, which is usually given simultaneously with salbutamol.

Oxygen therapy

Patients with acute asthma die from respiratory failure secondary to hypoxia. There is no indication of a primary cardiac event being involved. Based on this, patients with acute asthma should receive oxygen therapy. One systematic review showed no benefit from the use of a combination of helium and oxygen in acute asthma.

In a recent RCT it was shown that patients who received controlled oxygen therapy with fractional inspired oxygen (FiO_2) of 28% achieved better outcomes than patients treated with 100% oxygen. It would therefore appear

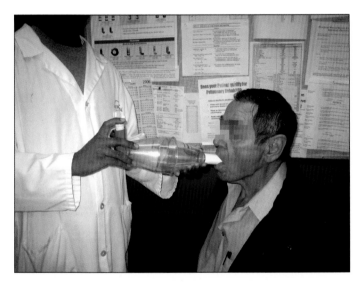

9.10 Patients may use a spacer device to increase the efficiency of the delivery of inhaled medication.

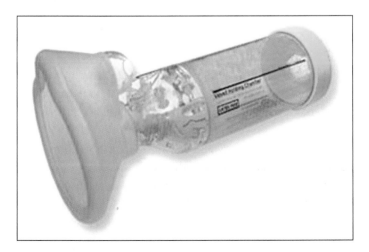

9.11 An example of a paediatric spacer device.

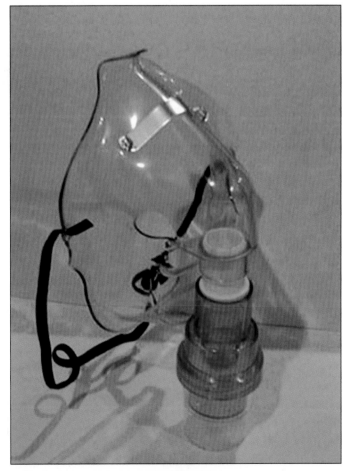

9.12 A face mask and nebulizer which can be used to deliver inhaled asthma medication.

reasonable to provide controlled oxygen therapy with ongoing oximetry and aim to achieve an oxygen saturation of greater than 90%.

Theophylline

There is no role for the routine use of aminophylline in acute asthma. A systematic review has found that it confers no additional bronchodilator effect to the routine use of inhaled bronchodilators.

Systemic corticosteroids

The role of systemic corticosteroids has been evaluated in two systematic reviews and one subsequent RCT. The first review found that early use of systemic corticosteroids (oral, intravenous, or intramuscular) versus placebo in the emergency department significantly reduced hospital admissions (OR 0.47; 95% CI 0.27 to 0.79; $P > 0.72$). The second review compared systematic steroids (intramuscular or oral) versus placebo after discharge from the emergency department. It found that systemic corticosteroids significantly reduced relapse at 7–10 days and hospital readmissions within 7 days compared with placebo (relapse rates five RCTs; 345 people; RR 0.35; 95% CI 0.17 to 0.73; hospital readmissions 4 RCTs; 210 people; RR 0.32; 95% CI 0.11 to 0.94). In addition, this review found no difference between oral and parenteral corticosteroids. A subsequent paediatric study, in which 30–60 mg (depending on age) of oral corticosteroids versus placebo were given in the emergency room or outpatient department, found that oral prednisone significantly reduced hospital admission rate compared with placebo (37/140 [26%] with prednisone *vs* 50/119 [42%] with placebo, $P > 0.01$).

There appears to be no difference in outcome for patients who do not taper the medicine versus those who taper their prednisone as long as the patient is taking regular inhaled corticosteroids as maintenance treatment. One RCT (20 people) compared 1 week with 2 weeks of oral prednisone after a 3-day course of intravenous methylprednisone and found no difference in PEFR and relapse rates. As these two studies were relatively small, treatment decisions should be individualized, based on patient's adherence and severity of asthma. The usual dose is 1 mg/kg to a maximum of 50 mg, which can conveniently be given as a single 50 mg tablet. Intravenous formulations should be considered only if there are concerns regarding drug absorption of oral medications because of vomiting, etc.

Inhaled steroids

Two systematic reviews have evaluated this intervention as well as two subsequent RCTs. The first review combined four paediatric studies. The second review, consisting mostly of adult patients, compared oral corticosteroids (prednisone) with high-dose inhaled corticosteroids >2 mg/day beclometasone dipropionate or equivalent) in people with acute asthma after emergency department discharge. It found no significant difference between oral and inhaled steroids for relapse rate at 7–10 days (OR relapse 1.00; 95% CI 0.66 to 1.52). In a more recent, well-designed study, Rodrigo evaluated 106 patients who received either fluticasone (3000 μg/h administered through a metered dose inhaler and spacer at 10-minute intervals for 3 hours, or 500 mg of intravenous hydrocortisone. All patients received standard doses of both salbutamol and ipratropium bromide. Patients treated with fluticasone showed 30.5% and 46.4% greater improvements in PEF and FEV_1, respectively, compared with the hydrocortisone group. The fluticasone group had better PEF and FEV_1 at 120, 150, and 180 minutes ($P < 0.05$). Also, the patients in the fluticasone group were more likely to be discharged, with the greatest benefit shown in those patients with the most severe obstruction. Subjects with a baseline FEV_1 of less than 11 treated with fluticasone showed a significant increase in pulmonary function ($P = 0.001$) and a significant decrease in hospitalization rate ($P = 0.05$). Although cost is a consideration, in countries where there is greater access to inhaled corticosteroids and the costs of acute asthma, especially hospitalizations, are significant, this may be a cost-effective intervention.

Magnesium

The initial rationale for the use of magnesium in acute asthma was based on the assumption that it might improve bronchodilatation. One systematic review and subsequent RCTs have shown no benefit (in terms of bronchodilatation) from the routine use of intravenous magnesium. In the systematic review, there was no significant difference between intravenous magnesium sulphate and placebo in hospital admissions (admission rates: OR 0.31; 95% CI 0.09 to 1.02). In a subgroup analysis the authors found that in patients presenting with an FEV_1 <30% at presentation, failure to respond to initial treatment, or failure to improve beyond 60% in FEV_1 after 1 h was associated with a significantly improved PEF volume and reduced rates of hospital admission compared with placebo (hospital admission rates: OR 0.10; 95% CI 0.04 to 0.27). Another RCT that included

42 patients who received both inhaled bronchodilators and intravenous corticosteroids, found that intravenous magnesium sulphate significantly improved PEFR at 60 minutes compared with placebo but had no effect on rates of hospitalizations. One subsequent RCT found no significant difference in hospital admissions between intravenous magnesium sulphate and placebo (18% with magnesium sulphate vs 25% with placebo; RR 0.71; 95% CI 0.19 to 2.67). Another RCT of 248 adults with an FEV_1 >30% predicted, all of whom were treated with methylprednisone and nebulized salbutamol found that 2 g of intravenous magnesium sulphate significantly improved lung function at 4 hours but had no impact on admission rates with 39/122 (32%) given magnesium sulphate vs 41/126 (32%) given placebo being admitted.

Discharge planning

Patient management should be individualized, so, for example, a patient who fails to improve as an outpatient on oral prednisone or who has a history of near-fatal asthma may require a more cautious approach. The majority of patients seen in the emergency department will be discharged. In general, patients who achieve 60% of their predicted or known best lung function can be safely discharged. Most patients should continue on oral corticosteroids and there is evidence that a combination of an inhaled corticosteroid is more effective than systemic corticosteroids alone.

Follow-up

Patients who have experienced an asthma exacerbation are at risk of subsequent exacerbations. It is clear that all patients benefit from an education programme and that facilitated referral to specialist care is also associated with better outcomes. It should be noted that adherence to medications prescribed on discharge is poor with a recent study showing that a significant proportion of patients discontinue both oral as well as inhaled corticosteroids in the days after discharge from hospital. Thus patients who have had an asthma exacerbation should not be left without appropriate follow-up and evaluation. Both how the patient responded to the development of the asthma exacerbation as well as the maintenance treatment the patient was on should be reassessed. If the patient was not already taking maintenance anti-inflammatory therapy this should be initiated and if the exacerbation occurred despite such therapy consideration should be given to increasing the dose and/or adding a long-acting β-agonist as maintenance therapy. This latter treatment has been associated with a reduction in the risk of asthma exacerbations when compared with increasing the dose of inhaled corticosteroids. In addition, previous recommendations to double the dose of inhaled corticosteroids early in an asthma exacerbation have recently been found to be ineffective and it is likely that at least a quadrupling of the dose of inhaled corticosteroids is required. This latter recommendation is based on emergency room studies, which have shown that quadrupling the usual dose of inhaled corticosteroids is equivalent to prednisone 40 mg, orally.

Summary

Exacerbations of asthma are a common medical emergency and one often managed suboptimally. Patients should be evaluated for historical factors for identifying high-risk patients. Assessment of the current exacerbation should include an objective assessment of airflow obstruction, in conjunction with the initiation of therapy with controlled oxygen therapy, regular bronchodilator therapy and in most cases systemic corticosteroids. A single 50 mg oral dose of prednisone is appropriate and there is no benefit in the use of intravenous corticosteroids. Ipratropium bromide may provide additional bronchodilator effect and, as with the use of intravenous magnesium, both therapies have been shown to reduce hospitalizations for moderate to severe exacerbations. Intravenous aminophylline or β-agonists have no role in the routine management of patients presenting with acute asthma. Patients who achieve 60% of their predicted PEF or FEV_1 or better can usually be safely discharged.

At the time of the exacerbation the opportunity should be taken to review how a patient responded, especially in the early stages of the attack. Specific issues should include whether they were on appropriate anti-inflammatory therapy, whether they modified the dose, or treatment, early in the exacerbation and also whether they had an action plan. Where deficiencies are identified, these can usually be corrected by a facilitated referral to a specialist clinic which ideally has an asthma education programme. Long-term treatment strategies as well as asthma education can be addressed at that time and, in particular, the need for long-term anti-inflammatory treatment as well as the potential incremental benefit of the addition of add-on therapy, most likely the use of a long-acting β-agonist, can be decided.

Conclusions

Asthma with appropriate maintenance therapy, a programme of asthma education and especially one that integrates a written action plan will be associated with a reduced risk of asthma exacerbations. In the absence of, or despite these strategies, patients will suffer acute asthma exacerbations. Management should involve a concise history focusing on the immediate precipitating factors as well as historical risk factors. Treatment for most patients will involve regular bronchodilator therapy, systemic corticosteroids and potentially the addition of inhaled corticosteroids acutely and magnesium for more severe attacks. All patients should receive education and appropriate follow-up to evaluate the events leading up to the exacerbation and the development of a strategy to prevent future exacerbations.

Further reading

Awadh N, Grunfeld A, FitzGerald JM (1999). Health care costs associated with acute asthma. A prospective economic analysis. *Can Respir J*, **6**:521–525.

Carruthers DM, Harrison BD (1995). Arterial blood gas analysis or oxygen saturation in the assessment of acute asthma? *Thorax*, **50**:186–188.

FitzGerald JM, Becker A, Sears MR, Mink S, Chung K, Lee J; Canadian Asthma Exacerbation Study Group (2004). A randomized controlled trial of doubling the dose of inhaled corticosteroids versus placebo in acute asthma exacerbations. *Thorax*, **59**:550–556.

FitzGerald JM, Gibson P (2006). Asthma exacerbations: prevention. *Thorax*, **61**:992–999.

Gibson PG, Powell H, Coughlan J, Wilson AJ, Abramson M, Haywood P, Bauman A, Hensley MJ, Walters EH (2003). Self-management education and regular practitioner review for adults with asthma. *Cochrane Database Syst Rev*, **1**:CD001117.

Global strategy for asthma (1995). Management and Prevention. NIH Publication No 02–3659. Online (http://www.ginasthma.com/Guidelineitem.asp).

Masoli M, Fapian D, Holt S, Beasly R (2004). Global burden of asthma. A report developed for the Global Initiative for Asthma. Global Initiative for Asthma, Online (http://www.ginasthma.com).

Mountain RD, Heffner JE, Brackett NC, Jr, Sahn SA (1990). Acid base disturbances in acute asthma. *Chest*, **98**:651–55.

Nowak RM, Tomlanovich MC, Sarkar DD, Kvale PA, Anderson JA (1983). Arterial blood gases and pulmonary function testing in acute bronchial asthma. *JAMA*, **246**:2043–2046.

Rodrigo GJ, Rodrigo C (1993). Assessment of the patient with acute asthma in the emergency department. A factor analytic study. *Chest*, **104**:1325–1328.

Rodrigo GJ, Rodrigo C, Burschtin O (1999). Ipratropium bromide in acute adult severe asthma: a meta-analysis of randomized controlled trials. *Am J Med*, **107**:363–370.

Rodrigo GJ (2005). Comparison of inhaled fluticasone with intravenous hydrocortisone in the treatment of adult acute asthma. *Am J Respir Crit Care Med*, **171**:1231–1236.

Rodrigo GJ, Rodrigo C, Hall JB (2004). Acute asthma in adults: a review. *Chest*, **125**:1081–1102.

Rowe BH, Bretzlaff JA, Bourdon C, Bota GW, Camargo CA Jr (2002). Magnesium sulphate for treating exacerbations of acute asthma in the emergency department. In: *Cochrane Database Syst Rev*, **3**:CD001490.

Rowe BH, Spooner CH, Ducharme FM, Bretzlaff JA, Bota GW (2002). Corticosteroids for preventing relapse following acute exacerbations of asthma. In: *Cochrane Database Syst Rev*, **3**:CD000195.

Shim CS, Williams MH, Jr (1983). Relationship of wheezing to the severity of obstruction in asthma. *Arch Intern Med*, **143**:890–892.

Stein LM, Cole RP (1990). Early administration of corticosteroids in emergency room treatment of acute asthma. *Ann Intern Med*, **112**:822–827.

Turner M, Patel A, Ginsberg S, FitzGerald JM (1997). Bronchodilator therapy in acute airflow obstruction: a meta-analysis. *Arch Intern Med*, **157**:1736–1744.

Turner MO, Noertjojo K, Vedal S, Bai T, Crump S, Fitzgerald JM (1998). Risk factors for near-fatal asthma. A case-control study in hospitalized patients with asthma. *Am J Respir Crit Care Med*, **157**:1804.

Zieverink SE, Harper AP, Holden RW, Klatte EC, Brittain H (1982). Emergency room radiography of asthma: an efficacy study. *Radiology*, **145**:27–29.

Chapter 10

Paediatric Asthma

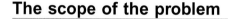

Sejal Saglani, Elizabeth Biggart and Andrew Bush

The scope of the problem

Coughing and wheezing is common in childhood; in Tucson, 50% of children will have wheezed at least once before their sixth birthday, and the ISAAC study suggests more than 30% of British teenagers have asthma. Many of the reported symptoms are trivial, and either unrelated to asthma or require minimal treatment. It appears also that the rate of rise of true asthma prevalence is flattening off. Nonetheless, it is still the fact that children are being over- and under-diagnosed with asthma.

Definition

The simplest definition, which is what has to be relied on in clinical practice, is that of the International Consensus Group: 'cough and/or wheeze in a setting where asthma is likely, and other rare causes have been excluded'. The great merit of this definition is that it makes no assumptions about underlying pathology and therefore the most appropriate treatment. To this definition we would add for consideration:

- Unless there is significant *breathlessness* there is unlikely to be significant asthma.
- In older children, there is evidence of variable airflow obstruction (usually but not always peak flow) over time and with treatment.
- In younger children, the definition could encompass a response to asthma treatment, with relapse on cessation of treatment and a second response when treatment is re-instituted.

Diagnosis of asthma in childhood

The majority of children will be diagnosed solely on the basis of the history and physical examination. Specific points which should lead to suspicion that the problem is more than just asthma are listed in *Tables 10.1* and *10.2*, respectively.

An approach to differential diagnosis is given in *Table 10.3*. Of note are the following:

- Wheeze is used ambiguously by children and families, and the statement 'my child wheezes' should never be accepted uncritically.
- If symptoms have truly started on the first day of life, then the diagnosis is not asthma, and congenital malformations or primary ciliary dyskinesia should be considered.

Table 10.1 Points to seek in the history suggesting a different or supplementary diagnosis

- Are the child/family really describing wheeze?
- Upper airway symptoms – snoring, rhinitis, sinusitis
- Symptoms from the first day of life
- Very sudden onset of symptoms
- Chronic moist cough/sputum production
- Worse wheeze or irritable after feed, worse when lying down, vomiting, choking on feeds
- Any feature of a systemic immunodeficiency
- Continuous, unremitting or worsening symptoms
- Symptoms which disappear when the child is asleep

Table 10.2 Points to seek in the physical examination suggesting a different or supplementary diagnosis

- Digital clubbing, signs of weight loss, failure to thrive
- Upper airway disease – enlarged tonsils and adenoids, prominent rhinitis, nasal polyps
- Unusually severe chest deformity (Harrison's sulcus, barrel chest)
- Fixed monophonic wheeze
- Stridor (monophasic or biphasic)
- Asymmetrical wheeze
- Signs of cardiac or systemic disease

Table 10.3 Differential diagnosis of asthma in childhood

- Upper airway disease – adenotonsillar hypertrophy, rhinosinusitis, post-nasal drip
- Congenital structural bronchial disease – complete cartilage rings, cysts, webs
- Bronchial/tracheal compression – vascular rings and pulmonary artery sling, enlarged cardiac chamber; lymph nodes enlarged by tuberculosis or lymphoma
- Endobronchial disease – foreign body, tumour
- Oesophageal/swallowing problems – gastro-oesophageal reflux, inco-ordinate swallow, laryngeal cleft or H-type tracheo-oesophageal fistula
- Causes of pulmonary suppuration – cystic fibrosis, primary ciliary dyskinesia, any systemic immunodeficiency including agammaglobulinaemia, severe combined immunodeficiency
- Psychological – vocal cord dysfunction, hyperventilation
- Miscellaneous – bronchopulmonary dysplasia, congenital or acquired tracheomalacia, pulmonary oedema secondary to left to right shunting, or cardiomyopathy

- The history of aspiration of a foreign body (**10.1**) may not be volunteered, and should be specifically sought. Clues include sudden onset of symptoms and asymmetrical physical signs.
- Cystic fibrosis is not just a diagnosis of childhood; beware of 'asthma plus', another suspicious feature such as nasal polyps (**10.2**), rectal prolapse or failure to thrive.
- The child with a chronic (>6 weeks) productive cough may have bronchiectasis not asthma, and should be referred for investigation.
- Symptoms which completely disappear during sleep are likely due to functional problems such as vocal cord dysfunction (**10.3**).
- If there is no atopic history (eczema, food allergy), the diagnosis of airway inflammation causing asthma should be reconsidered. In cases of doubt, skin prick tests might be obtained.

In addition, simple investigations may be performed in the minority of children, such as a chest X-ray. However, many important diagnoses, including foreign body and cystic fibrosis, are still possible despite normal X-ray findings.

In addition, in older children (usually age 5 years or more), the following tests should be considered to try to document variable airflow obstruction:

- response of peak flow acutely to a β_2-agonist administered via a spacer

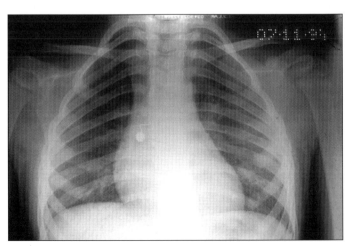

10.1 Endobronchial foreign body. There is a nose stud in the right bronchus intermedius.

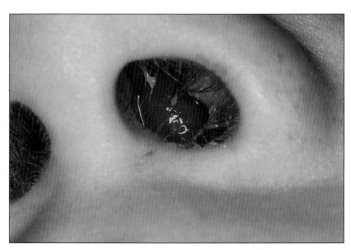

10.2 The child's left nostril is almost completely occluded by a large polyp, typical of cystic fibrosis.

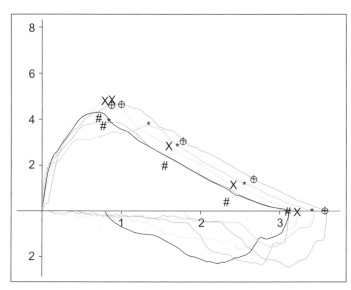

10.3 Flow volume curve showing normal expiratory loop (above the horizontal axis), but marked impairment of inspiratory flow due to adduction of the vocal cords.

- home peak flow monitoring for 2 weeks
- response of peak flow to a simple screening exercise test (can be made more rigorous in special centres)
- (special centres only) response to inhaled methacholine challenge.

A normal test does not exclude asthma, but the more of these tests that fail to document variable airflow obstruction, the less likely is asthma. *Perhaps the single most common diagnostic mistake in the older child is the failure to document variable airflow obstruction prior to making a diagnosis of asthma.* If

doubt remains, and particularly in young children, a therapeutic trial should be considered:

- Commence moderate dose inhaled steroid for 6–12 weeks; if there is no response, the child can be assumed not to have steroid responsive asthma.
- If there appears to be a 'response', *stop the treatment* (this is the absolutely key step, otherwise children with transient, spontaneously resolving symptoms will be labelled as 'asthma'.
- Only diagnose asthma if symptoms recur, and respond again to inhaled steroids, in which case the dose is tapered to the lowest needed to control symptoms.

Wheezing phenotypes in early childhood

There are many causes of wheeze in the pre-school years, and not all respond to inhaled steroids (*Table 10.4*). In real life, there is of course overlap between phenotypes, but it is useful to consider them as a guide to group mechanisms, and also when individualizing an asthma treatment plan. Of particular note are three types, with very different courses (**10.4**):

- Transient wheeze – onset before age 3 years, with disappearance of symptoms by age 6, usually non-atopic, and symptoms with viral colds.
- Persistent wheeze – onset before age 3 years, symptoms still present at 6 years, usually atopic, symptoms often initially just with viral colds, but then symptoms between colds with typical triggers.
- Late-onset wheeze – symptoms between age 3 and 6 years, non-atopic.

A current debate is whether infection with respiratory syncytial virus (RSV) causes later asthma or atopy. If it does, it must interact with other factors, since RSV infection is almost universal in the first 2 years of life. It is clear that atopic children are more likely to have severe RSV infections, but evidence from prospective studies is that children who get RSV bronchiolitis have abnormal pre-morbid lung function, which tracks into mid-childhood (**10.5**). Whether there are also pre-existing immunological abnormalities is less clear. The best follow-up data, with complete ascertainment, is from Tucson, and is reassuring that, although there are persistent symptoms, these gradually improve, and RSV does not cause asthma (**10.6**).

Table 10.4 The different phenotypes of wheeze in the pre-school years

Pre-school asthma syndrome	Inflammatory component	Extent of BHR	Extent of PAL
Chronic lung disease of prematurity	? (probably none)	+	+ (antenatal onset)
Post-bronchiolitis (e.g. post respiratory syncytial virus infection)	? (probably none)	+	+ (antenatal onset)
Virus-associated wheeze	–	–	+ (antenatal onset)
Atopy-associated wheeze	+ (probably often eosinophilic)	+	+ (probably antenatal and post-natal onset)
Obliterative bronchiolitis (e.g. post adenoviral infection)	–	–	+ (post-natal onset)
Non-atopy associated, later-onset wheeze	?present, ?type	Probably present	+ (probably at least post-natal onset)

BHR, bronchial hyper-reactivity; PAL, persistent airflow limitation.

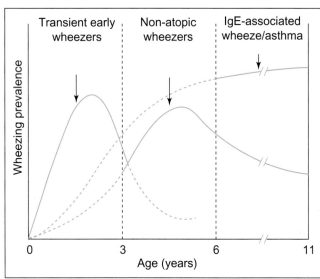

10.4 The different wheezing phenotypes in childhood. Transient early wheezers are symptomatic in the first three years of life, but stop wheezing by age 6 years. They are typically non-atopic. The IgE-associated wheezers have symptoms persisting into childhood. In practice, these phenotypes are often only diagnosable retrospectively. Redrawn with permission from Stein RT (1997). Peak flow variability, methacholine responsiveness and atopy as markers for detecting different wheezing phenotypes in childhood. *Thorax*, **52**:946–952.

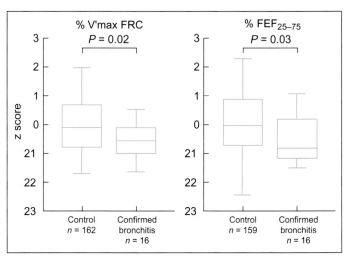

10.5 Lung function before and after bronchiolitis. The group of children who went on to develop acute bronchiolitis had reduced lung function (V'max FRC) prior to the illness; their reduced lung function tracked into mid-childhood. Note lung function is expressed as z scores. Redrawn with permission from Turner SW (2002). Reduced lung function both before bronchiolitis and at 11 years. *Arch Dis Child*, **87**:417–420.

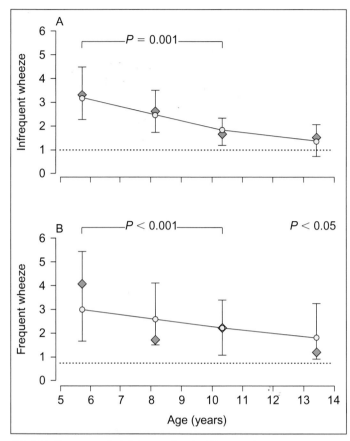

10.6 Follow-up of children who had a respiratory syncytial virus infection. Symptoms gradually improve over the years, and there is no increased prevalence of asthma. Redrawn with permission from Stein RT (1999). Respiratory syncytial virus in early life and risk of wheeze and allergy by age 13 years. *Lancet*, **354**:541–545.

Follow-up studies of the different wheezing phenotypes

No cohort study has recruited children antenatally and followed them through to death many decades later. Therefore, conclusions have to be based on overlapping cohort studies to attempt to build up a coherent lifetime picture. There are many such cohorts, which have provided different information, and space allows only a few to be summarized. The Tucson cohort has taught us (**10.7**):

- Transient wheezers have impaired lung function at birth, and although there is some catch-up, lung function remains impaired at age 16 years.

- Persistent wheezers have normal lung function at birth, but airflow obstruction by age 6 years, which tracks to age 16.
- Late-onset wheezers have normal lung function throughout.

From the Melbourne and other cohorts we have learned that for all phenotypes (atopic, virus-associated), lung function tracks from early childhood (age 7) into middle age (50 years old) (**10.8**). There are two important sources on the late consequences of these different phenotypes:

- The Aberdeen group has shown that people who had atopic asthma, but not 'wheezy bronchitis' (which we would now call transient wheeze, or virus-associated wheeze) have a reduction in spirometry in middle age compared with normals, but the rate of deterioration (ageing) of spirometry is equal, and faster in both groups than normal (**10.9**).

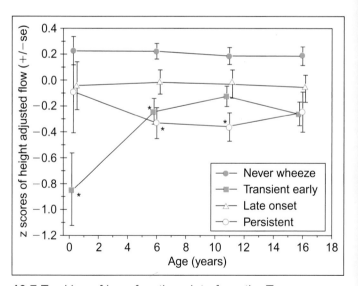

10.7 Tracking of lung function: data from the Tucson cohort. The transient early wheezers are born with low lung function, which has improved, albeit not to normal, by age 6; thereafter, there is no catch-up growth. The persistent wheezers, are normal at birth, have airflow obstruction by age 6, and thereafter lung function tracks. The late-onset wheezers do not show any decrement of lung function. Reproduced with permission from Morgan WJ *et al.* (2005). Outcome of asthma and wheezing in the first 6 years of life: follow-up through adolescence. *Am J Respir Crit Care Med*, **172**:1253–1258.

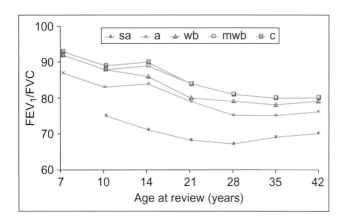

10.8 Data from the Melbourne cohort. Tracking of lung function from childhood into middle-age, irrespective of wheeze phenotype. c, control; mwb, mild wheezy bronchitis (wheezy bronchitis would today probably be called virus-associated wheeze); wb, wheezy bronchitis; a, asthma; sa, severe asthma. FEV_1, forced expiratory volume in one second; FVC, forced vital capacity. Reproduced with permission from Oswald H *et al.* (1997). Childhood asthma and lung function in mid-adult life. *Pediatr Pulmonol*, **23**:14–20.

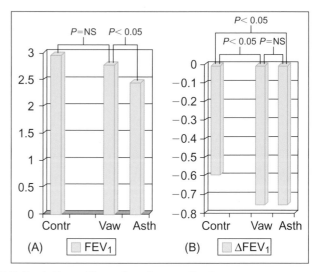

10.9 Evolution of lung function as the lung ages (data from Aberdeen). The patients were recruited in childhood, and studied at around age 50 years. The virus-associated wheezers (Vaw) attain the same lung function (forced expiratory volume in one second [FEV_1]) as controls, but asthmatic patients (Asth) have reduced FEV_1 (**A**). However (**B**) the Vaw and asthmatic patients are losing FEV_1 at the same rate, and faster than the normal controls. Redrawn from Edwards CA *et al.* (2003). Wheezy bronchitis in childhood: a distinct clinical entity with lifelong significance? *Chest*, **124**:18–24.

- Barker's group, using death certificate data, have shown that, over a wide range of communities, there is a strong correlation between the mortality rate in that area for infant pneumonia and bronchitis and the standardized mortality rate for chronic bronchitis and emphysema 50 years later (**10.10**).

Thus putting these data together into a consistent model, it would appear that something happens before birth (virus-associated wheezers) or in the first 6 years of life (atopic asthmatics) which produces airway obstruction. There is then no 'catch-up' growth throughout adult life. When the lungs start to age, these people have an accelerated ageing pattern, making them more prone to chronic obstructive pulmonary disease. Thus, early life events are of great importance if interventions are to be made to prevent the development of persistent airflow limitation.

The pathological correlates of this wealth of epidemiological data have not been well worked out. It is clear from a number of studies that at least one hallmark of adult asthma, thickening of the reticular basement membrane, is present to the same degree in children with asthma (**10.11**). Recent work has shown that atopic infants at a year of age, with symptoms and bronchodilator reversibility, do not have structural airway wall changes (**10.12**). Thus, at some time during the second to the fourth year of life, fixed changes develop. How best to prevent this is unknown.

Early life events: why do pre-school children wheeze?

The 'cause' of asthma is elusive, but a number of studies have suggested important issues, some of which are summarized below:

Genetic factors

The quest for an 'asthma gene' has led to numerous studies in which the identification of a gene has been followed rapidly by a further study which has failed to replicate the finding. This is perhaps unsurprising, since genes exert their effect in the context of an environment and, increasingly, the importance of studying the two together has been appreciated.

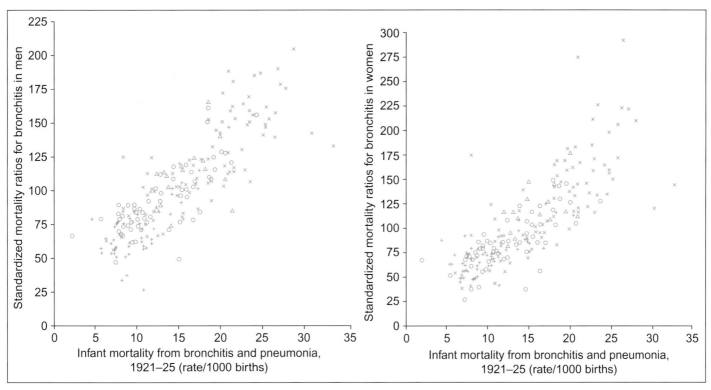

10.10 Relationship between early death from infant respiratory disease, and subsequent standardized mortality rate for chronic bronchitis and emphysema: (**A**) men and (**B**) women. A high infant mortality rate over a range of communities is associated with a high subsequent mortality in the same area from chronic obstructive airway disease. Reproduced with permission from Barker DP (1993). *Fetal and Infant Origins of Adult Disease*. BMA Press, London. + = county boroughs, ○ = urban areas, × = rural areas △ = London boroughs.

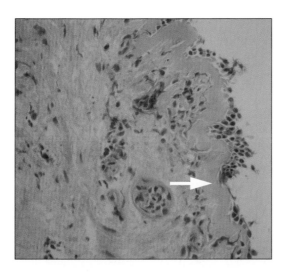

10.11 Haematoxylin and eosin stain of a severely thickened reticular basement membrane (arrow) from a 3-year-old asthmatic child.

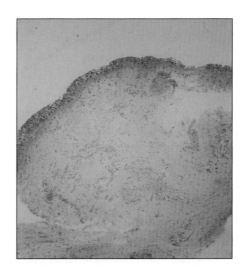

10.12 Endobronchial biopsy from a 1-year-old atopic infant with chronic wheeze, stained with toluidine blue. In contrast, there is no inflammation and no thickening of the reticular basement membrane.

Antenatal factors

Airway obstruction is present very shortly after birth in the infants of mothers who are atopic, or who smoke during pregnancy, or have hypertension of pregnancy. There is evidence that this fixed airflow obstruction persists (above). The exact mechanism is unclear, but may involve loss of alveolar tethering to the airways, leading to a passive reduction in calibre. Illustrating the importance of gene–environment interactions is the finding that the effects of cigarette smoke on lung function are seen in mothers who have the null polymorphism for glutathione-S-transferase, an enzyme which is involved in defence against oxidants.

Postnatal factors

The 'hygiene hypothesis' has generated huge research interest. The original observations, which are simple and incontestable, are that atopy becomes less common the more older siblings there are in the family. The interpretation of the observation has proved much more challenging. First, it should be noted that atopy and asthma are not the same thing, and prevalences of the two may vary independently worldwide. Originally, on the basis of observations on early infection and asthma, it was suggested that early recurrent viral infections are the important factor. Certainly, first-born children, but not subsequent children, placed in a child care facility in the first year of life have more wheezing illnesses early on, but less after age 6 years. This was attributed to the early acquisition of multiple viral infections from other children. More recently, the observation that there is a low prevalence of asthma in children born on farms has focused attention on other possibilities, including early exposure to endotoxin. The complexities of gene–environment interactions has been shown in this context. A meta-analysis suggested that CD14 was not a gene involved in asthma. However, in a much more detailed and focused study, the CD 14/-260 C→T polymorphism in the CD14 promoter was associated with higher levels of both total and specific immunoglobulin (Ig)E to aeroallergens in children in regular contact with domestic pets, but the opposite relationship, not explained by endotoxin levels, in children in contact with stable animals, an example of so-called phenotypic plasticity, whereby the operation of a gene can be radically different depending on the environment of the organism.

Primary prevention?

At the moment, we know that encouraging breastfeeding, and keeping children away from cigarette smoke exposure are good things to do. In terms of allergens, we do not know whether to reduce or increase exposure in early life, to try to prevent sensitization or induce high zone tolerance respectively. Certainly, some attempts at reducing allergen exposure have actually been counterproductive, leading to an increase in allergen sensitization. What is not controversial is that allergens to which the child is already sensitized should be excluded from the environment where possible.

Treatment of paediatric asthma

Recent detailed evidence-based guidelines have been issued, detailing a step-up and step-down approach to therapy. Inevitably, in children the evidence base is much less than in adults, and least of all in young infants.

Environmental issues

There are important aspects to consider before reaching for the prescription pad. These are:

- Is there passive smoke exposure? Active smoke exposure leads to relative steroid resistance, and there are many mechanisms whereby environmental tobacco smoke adversely interacts with asthma therapy.
- Is the child sensitized and exposed to high doses of allergens? Even if allergen exposure is insufficient to cause acute deterioration, it may cause secondary steroid resistance by an interleukin (IL)-2 and IL-4 dependent mechanism. Exposure to cat allergen at school from the clothes of pet-owning peers may be sufficient to cause asthma in cat allergic children to deteriorate during the school week, improving at the weekend and during school holidays.

Drug delivery device issues

Part of the routine of the paediatric asthma clinic is a check on inhaler technique, usually by an experienced respiratory nurse. Errors are common, and repeated instruction may be necessary if a good technique is to be achieved (**10.13**). A choice of spacers and other devices should be offered (**10.14**). The age-appropriate choices for inhaler devices are summarized in *Table 10.5*. If a metered dose inhaler and spacer is used, some simple rules should be followed:

- The inhaler should be shaken between each activation.

- There should be no delay between activating the spacer into the spacer and the mask being applied to the child's face.
- If the child is crying, he or she will take big inspirations, but drug deposition in the lower airway will be exactly zero.
- Unless a metal spacer is used, when this is unnecessary, electrostatic deposition of medication to the side of the spacer can be reduced by cleaning it with soapy water once per week, and leaving it to drain; rinsing and rubbing dry should be avoided.

A nebulizer is only indicated in the most severe cases of acute asthma; if it must be used, a tight-fitting mask is essential;

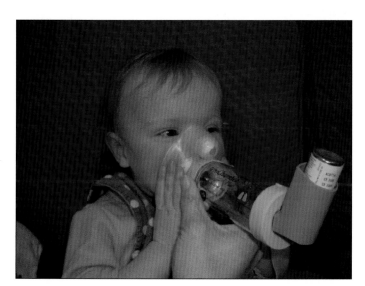

10.13 Toddler using an aerochamber and bronchodilator. Note that the child is calm, not crying, and the mask is gently but firmly applied over the nose and mouth.

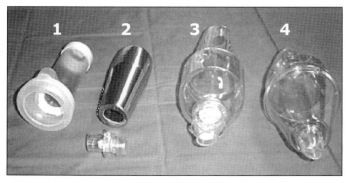

10.14 Commonly used spacers. 1, Aerochamber; 2, Nebuchamber; 3, Nebuhaler; 4, Volumatic.

there is no use holding the cup close to the child's face and hoping for the best.

Treatment of the pre-school asthmatic child

Stepwise guidelines have been proposed, with treatment escalating if there is no response to treatment. Perhaps insufficient attention has been given to different phenotypes (above). For example, symptoms with viral colds, in a non-atopic child with no symptoms between colds, would logically be treated with intermittent high dose inhaled corticosteroids at the time of the viral cold, perhaps combined with an oral leukotriene receptor antagonist. Given the evidence that such children do not have eosinophilic inflammation between colds, and the poor response of viral cold-induced symptoms to prophylactic inhaled steroids, there is little logic in regular therapy. There is also little evidence that post-RSV symptoms respond to anything much, so blindly escalating useless treatment is futile. Atopic wheezers can be treated with low dose inhaled corticosteroids, with additional leukotriene receptor antagonists if response is unsatisfactory. If a child is non-responsive to escalating treatment, consider whether:

- the child does not have asthma at all (the younger the child, the more likely is an alternative diagnosis)
- the child has a non-steroid sensitive wheezing phenotype.

Also do not blindly and uncritically escalate therapy.

Treatment of asthma in the older child

The step-up and step-down guidelines are very similar to those in adults, although with less of an evidence base (**10.15**). It is important to remember that the natural history of asthma in childhood is for improvement, and at each clinic visit, if the child has been well controlled, then therapy should be tapered down.

Monitoring asthma in the clinic

Monitoring lung function

All children should have an age-appropriate lung function test at each clinic visit, usually spirometry. Some children as young as 2 years can use a spirometer with appropriate coaching and incentive software (**10.16**). Other devices, such as the interrupter technique, have still to find a place in the routine work of the clinic.

Table 10.5 Age-appropriate choices of asthma drug delivery devices

Age of child	Device	Considerations
Less than 2 years	Spacer with mask and metered dose inhaler (MDI)	Careful introduction to familiarize child with mask – *use of play*
More than 2 years	Spacer using mouthpiece; small spacers are convenient for patient	Once a child can keep lips round mouthpiece and breath through mouth – *praise and incentives*
More than 6 years	Dry powder device	Once a child is able to take a steady and deep inhalation and hold breath – *more praise*
More than 12 years	Breath-actuated MDI	Not ideal but may be better alternative to MDI alone as inhalation co-ordination can be a problem – *listen to young person*
At any age	Nebulizer	A nebulizer is only indicated in the most severe cases of acute asthma; if it must be used, a tight-fitting mask is essential; there is no use holding the cup close to the child's face and hoping for the best

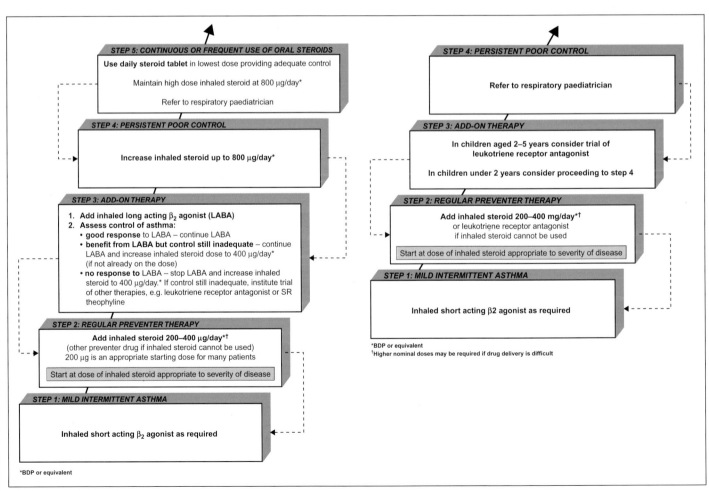

STEP 5: CONTINUOUS OR FREQUENT USE OF ORAL STEROIDS
Use daily steroid tablet in lowest dose providing adequate control
Maintain high dose inhaled steroid at 800 μg/day*
Refer to respiratory paediatrician

STEP 4: PERSISTENT POOR CONTROL
Increase inhaled steroid up to 800 μg/day*

STEP 3: ADD-ON THERAPY
1. **Add inhaled long acting β₂ agonist (LABA)**
2. **Assess control of asthma:**
 • **good response** to LABA – continue LABA
 • **benefit from LABA but control still inadequate** – continue LABA and increase inhaled steroid dose to 400 μg/day* (if not already on the dose)
 • **no response to LABA** – stop LABA and increase inhaled steroid to 400 μg/day.* If control still inadequate, institute trial of other therapies, e.g. leukotriene receptor antagonist or SR theophyline

STEP 2: REGULAR PREVENTER THERAPY
Add inhaled steroid 200–400 μg/day*†
(other preventer drug if inhaled steroid cannot be used)
200 μg is an appropriate starting dose for many patients
Start at dose of inhaled steroid appropriate to severity of disease

STEP 1: MILD INTERMITTENT ASTHMA
Inhaled short acting β₂ agonist as required

*BDP or equivalent

STEP 4: PERSISTENT POOR CONTROL
Refer to respiratory paediatrician

STEP 3: ADD-ON THERAPY
In children aged 2–5 years consider trial of leukotriene receptor antagonist
In children under 2 years consider proceeding to step 4

STEP 2: REGULAR PREVENTER THERAPY
Add inhaled steroid 200–400 mg/day*†
or leukotriene receptor antagonist
if inhaled steroid cannot be used
Start at dose of inhaled steroid appropriate to severity of disease

STEP 1: MILD INTERMITTENT ASTHMA
Inhaled short acting β2 agonist as required

*BDP or equivalent
†Higher nominal doses may be required if drug delivery is difficult

10.15 Stepwise guidelines.

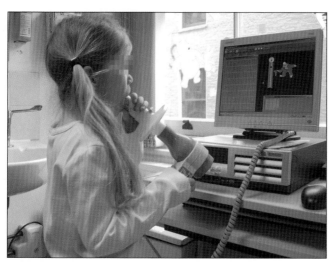

10.16 Child using incentive spirometry. On the screen is a clown and a bell on top of a pole. A maximal effort will lead to the bell being rung.

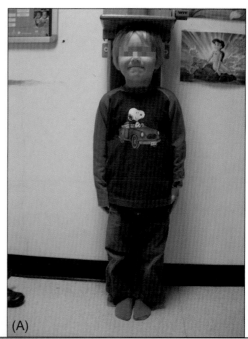

(A)

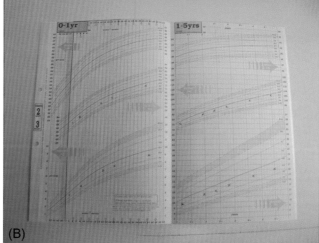

(B)

10.17A Child about to be measured using a Harpenden stadiometer.
10.17B Standard paediatric growth chart, with height and weight plotted. This is a mandatory requirement for all children being treated for asthma.

Monitoring growth

All children should have an accurate measurement of height and weight, which should be plotted on a growth chart (**10.17A,B**). Progress should be reviewed at each visit.

Monitoring inflammation

There is evidence that non-invasively monitoring inflammation using measurements of exhaled nitric oxide or induced sputum may improve outcome (**10.18A,B**). These measurements are currently confined to specialist centres.

Other monitoring

Children who are receiving very high dose (>800 µg/day budesonide equivalent) inhaled steroids should be considered for monitoring of adrenal function with a Synacthen test. If the child has been prescribed prolonged or multiple courses of oral steroids, then bone densitometry should be considered.

When should a child be referred for a second opinion?

- If the diagnosis is in doubt.
- If treatment at a reasonable level (and certainly, budesonide equivalent >800 µ/day) is not working.
- If any party (treating doctor, child, carer) is unhappy.

Severe asthma in childhood

By definition, children with severe asthma are insensitive to the doses of inhaled corticosteroids which normally successfully treat milder children. There are a number of causes to be considered. Key is to ask the right question, which is: What is it about this child, his environment, and his asthma that makes it difficult, not easy, to treat?

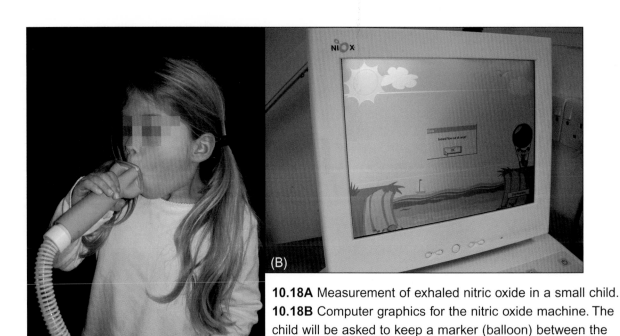

10.18A Measurement of exhaled nitric oxide in a small child.
10.18B Computer graphics for the nitric oxide machine. The child will be asked to keep a marker (balloon) between the two horizontal lines by blowing at the standardized flow rate.

Not asthma at all

Inhaled foreign body rarely responds to inhaled steroids; a full diagnostic review is mandatory.

Not taking the treatment

This may be because an inappropriate drug delivery device has been prescribed and the treatment cannot be taken, or more usually, for whatever reason, the child could take the therapy but does not do so. It is worth checking to see how many prescriptions have been collected from the general practitioner. Also, a depot injection of triamcinolone, which gives steroid cover for 4–6 weeks, may reveal that, if steroids are taken, the disease is sensitive!

If these two categories are eliminated, then we investigate children in a three-step protocol (**10.19**). After the first visit, some are allocated the label 'difficult asthma', because the root of the problem does not require any specially novel therapeutic approach.

Difficult asthma

Children in this category are sorted out at the first visit, which is a detailed multidisciplinary assessment, including:

- Skin prick tests, induced sputum, exhaled nitric oxide, spirometry with bronchodilator responsiveness.

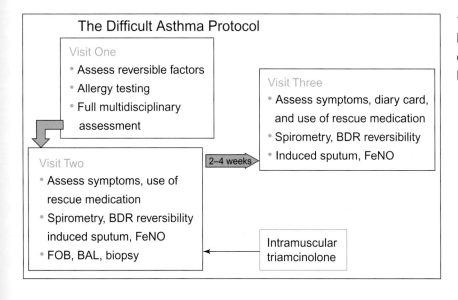

The Difficult Asthma Protocol

Visit One
- Assess reversible factors
- Allergy testing
- Full multidisciplinary assessment

Visit Two
- Assess symptoms, use of rescue medication
- Spirometry, BDR reversibility induced sputum, FeNO
- FOB, BAL, biopsy

2–4 weeks

Visit Three
- Assess symptoms, diary card, and use of rescue medication
- Spirometry, BDR reversibility
- Induced sputum, FeNO

Intramuscular triamcinolone

10.19 The difficult asthma protocol. BDR, bronchodilator; FeNO, fractional expired concentration of nitric oxide; FOB, fibre-optic bronchoscopy; BAL, bronchoalveolar lavage.

- Asthma nurse—home visit, school visit, checks inhaler technique, checks whether prescriptions have been issued.
- Clinical psychology assessment.
- ENT review of upper airway disease.

As a result of these assessments, reversible features are identified which means that asthma becomes controlled.

Really severe asthma

This group are investigated invasively, with a fibre-optic bronchoscopy, bronchoalveolar lavage, and endobronchial biopsy (**10.20**). While still under the anaesthetic, the child is given a single depot injection of triamcinolone. The response is assessed clinically, and with measurements of spirometry, exhaled nitric oxide and sputum induction. A number of different phenotypes have been proposed (*Table 10.6*), and

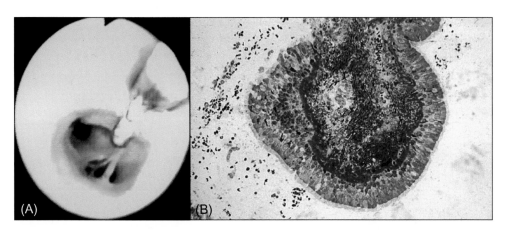

(A)   (B)

10.20 Performance of an endobronchial biopsy. (**A**) The forceps gripping a subcarina; (**B**) Typical biopsy obtained using a bronchoscope with a 2 mm channel.

Table 10.6 Phenotypes in really severe asthma in older children

Clinical scenario	Presumptive diagnosis	Suggested action
1. Continued airflow obstruction, no inflammation, no reversibility to β_2-agonists	Presumed obliterative bronchiolitis	• Inspiratory and expiratory computed tomography scan • Use minimum treatment which maintains lung function
2. Continued airflow obstruction, no inflammation, but with reversibility to β_2-agonists	Presumed steroid resistant, non-inflammatory bronchial reactivity	• Continuous subcutaneous terbutaline treatment
3. Persistent eosinophilic inflammation, with either or both of airflow obstruction and symptoms	Presumed steroid partial or complete resistance	• Look for causes of secondary steroid resistance • Treat with either prolonged high dose steroids or steroid-sparing agent
4. Persistent eosinophilic inflammation, with no airflow obstruction or symptoms	Possible lagging of clearance of inflammation	• Observe closely with repeated spirometry and non-invasive measures of inflammation
5. Presumed inflammation completely resolved with steroids (normal lung function, no symptoms)	Steroid sensitive asthma, but requiring high dose treatment	• Look for causes of secondary steroid resistance • Taper steroids to level at which symptoms are controlled without side effects, or use steroid-sparing agent
6. Persistent non-eosinophilic inflammation	Presumed other inflammatory mechanisms (other cells, e.g. neutrophilic inflammation; neurogenic mechanisms)	• Reduce steroid treatment to minimum level needed to control eosinophilic inflammation • Consider macrolides, or theophylline if neutrophilic inflammation

an individual treatment plan is developed. This is the really hard-core group which is the most difficult to treat, even with this detailed assessment. Therapeutic options include:

- cyclosporin for genuine steroid-resistant eosinophilic asthma
- macrolides for neutrophilic inflammation
- subcutaneous terbutaline (**10.21**) for persistent, non-inflammatory airway lability.

Conclusions

Early life events leading to asthma have a life-long effect on lung function. There are many wheezing phenotypes in childhood, and an individual treatment plan is necessary. This should include an assessment of environmental factors as well as drug delivery device. Treatment should be stepped down as soon as control has been achieved.

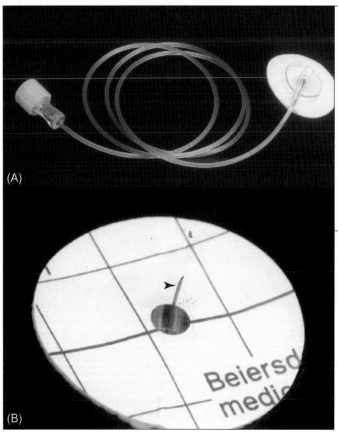

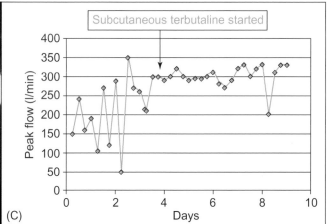

10.21 The use of subcutaneous terbutaline. (**A**) The giving set; (**B**) the needle ➤ used to attain subcutaneous access; and (**C**) a peak flow chart, showing a swinging peak flow stabilized by subcutaneous terbutaline. With thanks to Dr Donald Payne.

Further reading

British Guideline on the Management of Asthma (2003). *Thorax*, **58**(Suppl 1):S1–94.

Silverman M (2002). *Childhood Asthma and Other Wheezing Disorders*, 2nd edition. Arnold, London.

Index